Anthony Lawton

Fit to Care

Fit to Care

Editing, typesetting and publishing by UK Book Publishing

www.ukbookpublishing.com

ISBN: 978-1-917329-13-2

Contents

Fit to Care

Acknowledgements

One of my favourite quotes of all time is by Socrates, **"All I know is that I know nothing."** This will be referenced in several places throughout the book because it is so relevant, and by the end of this book, you will understand why. (Don't close the book just yet, Socrates was one of the smartest people who ever lived!)

This ongoing journey of learning (associated with this quote) keeps my love for life pumping through my veins. However, I understand why this makes me painful to live with! Therefore, I dedicate this book to my wife, Lyn, and my two sons, George, and Charlie, for always supporting me.

This book benefited hugely from the significant contributions of the 20 interviewed nurses.[1] Their insights, coming from various areas of the NHS[2], provided invaluable additional context and content. I am enormously grateful to them and give my sincerest thanks. Please also see "The Nurses Interviewed section". (*Please note, I have streamlined the nurse interview transcripts for brevity and clarity by removing things like "umm" and unrelated dialogue, as well as asides and conversational overlaps. I have not altered the meaning of anything said or put words in anyone's mouth.*)

In addition, this book was made possible due to the influence and inspiration from the professors and practitioners whose work I have studied and implemented over more than ten years. I am grateful to all of them for their valuable contributions to my knowledge.

I would also like to thank the NHS. For more than 16 years, I have worked with amazing people who, first and foremost, are wonderful human beings. Working with them, I have developed a comprehensive understanding of the following points linked to this book:

1. How far our society still has to go in reducing inequality. In that context, I hope that this book can make positive contributions to the deep-seated challenges of racism and the underrepresentation

---

1 Ranging in age from early 20s to late 60s, with a good mix of regional locations and a mix of ethnicities.

2 With experience in Primary Care, Secondary Care and Community Care.

of ethnic minority staff in senior positions within society, including the NHS.

2. Given that the nursing workforce is also predominantly female and with a higher proportion of older staff than other professions[3], this book also wishes to highlight the pivotal area of women's health issues; particularly menopause.

Academic Influencers:

Professor John Vervaeke, Professor Matthew Cripps, Professor John Seddon, Viktor Frankl, Patrick Lencioni, Dr BJ Fogg, Margaret Wheatley, Dr Robert Sapolsky

---

3 as of 2021/22, one in five professionals on the Nursing and Midwifery Council's (NMC) register are aged 56 or over, and almost one in ten are over 60, approaching retirement age (https://lordslibrary.parliament.uk/the-nursing-workforce-royal-college-of-nursing-report/)

Foreword

Conceptually, health and wellbeing in the workplace is nothing new, we have known for many decades that caring for colleagues or to coin an American phrase 'co-workers' can reap significant benefits for both the individual and the people, productivity, profit, and reputation. In nursing, our collective conscious can now be defined by two time periods related to one conspicuous pandemic, before COVID (bC) and after COVID (aC). The COVID pandemic brought into sharp focus the fragility of our health services and population health, yet despite what can arguably be described as the biggest health threat in our lifetime, nurses and the wider profession quietly, purposefully, and expertly saved a generation. It is true, we did this with others, we worked in collaboration, indeed one of the skills of a nurse is the ability to connect with other professions, families, and communities, but it was nurses, at the front, putting themselves in harm's way, stepping into the unknown, to save a generation. In thinking about our contribution to population health, be that in the home, a GP surgery, hospital ward, community clinic, in the air or on the sea, we seldom ever take the time to truly think about what it means to be 'Fit to Care', we are after all in service to others.

Through the 'lived experience' of 20 incredible nurses, 'Fit to Care' takes us on a journey of endeavour and discovery, a non-nursing view of the profession, through personal experiences and opportunities to work alongside nurses and the profession the author allows us to glimpse into their own 'lived experience' of connecting with the profession. It is hard not to have a romantic perception about the work of nurses and the nursing profession, through descriptive words such as 'love' and 'care' we get to understand the deep connection the author has with those exceptional nurses with the socially constructed X Factor traits. We know that modern day nursing practice has moved considerably from the preconceived images of 1970s, for it is now very much considered a 'safety critical' profession, an all-graduate profession, and a profession with established academic and scientific credentials. However, despite this progress, today the profession continues to be undermined by patriarchy, misogyny, sexism, racism, and a whole manner of discriminatory social norms, these individually and collectively contribute to demeaning the value of nursing and nurses.

Nursing work is deeply rewarding but is tough, from the 'cradle to the grave' is a poetic description of our work, but it is so much more than this, there are times when even I cannot describe what I am witness to, from the heroic efforts of a resuscitation room, to the quiet moments of a coaching conversation, nurses are the very essence of our way of life, they are the fabric that connects us in health and in illness, and in life and in death. The challenges for our profession are exciting, but enormous, the testimony of the 20 nurses brings to life the complex challenges we face today and tomorrow, not least our aging population, increasing acuity, societal expectations of healthcare, regulation, and the wider determinants of health, put together it's hard not to be intrigued by what the nursing profession can do tackle some of the greatest threats to society and its health.

Section one of 'Fit to Care' takes us on an unenviable journey into some of the challenges for nursing today, many of the macro pressures are as a direct result of geopolitics faced globally, many countries similar to the United Kingdom (UK) are facing an increasingly elderly population with increasing demand being placed on health and care services. Here in the UK, since the financial crisis in 2008, successive Governments have struggled to invest in public services, coupled with political indifference and the cost-of-living crisis, our society has steadily fragmented resulting in the increase of health inequalities, and for the first time in decades a reversal of life expectancy. The resultant impact of the cost-of-living crisis on our profession has been considerable, nurses are managing the complexity of communities who are unable to look after themselves, and as such have increasing health and care needs.

Leadership in nursing and the wider health and care professions is complex, most leaders, myself included, developed the art and science of leadership through 'trial and error', it is only in more recent times that the value of supporting clinical leaders has become popular, the range of NHS Leadership Academy programmes now offer an extensive range of options to support professional leadership. Like all leaders, we are inevitably answerable to someone, and like most Government targets they have broadly been driven by commitments made to the population, so in effect by electing a Government we give them the permission to deliver the standards (and targets) we would expect as a citizen. Leadership in nursing has changed significantly over the last 50 years, I have spent many an hour talking to my grandmother, a State Enrolled Nurse in the 1960s, about leadership, mostly through the prism of Matron, it is undeniable that this role was feared by most, yet in 2001, the then Government re-introduced the role of 'Modern Matron', in response to high profile care failures and issues with hospital cleanliness and discipline. Leadership and the value of leadership in nursing is a challenging construct, arguably all nurses are leaders, leading care for their patient or group of patients, leading teams, or leading services, each provides a progressive opportunity to ensure that nursing and nurses have a valid and valued seat at the table. All too often nurses are excluded, a case in example through the pandemic there was only one occasion when the Chief Nursing Officer for England was allowed at the nightly Government briefing; however, all NHS organisations have a nurse as a Board member, this is an important opportunity not only to advocate for the patients we care for, but also proactively and positively lead the profession. The nursing contribution at Board is often much more than about nursing, for nurses have and can make contributions beyond traditional practice environments, supporting operational delivery, financial stewardship, workforce transformation and strategy. Sometimes, leadership is about owning the space, being confident and supported to advance your ideas, and being courageous and brave in order to chart a new course if you feel that decisions are likely to cause harm.

Diversity, Equity, Inclusion, and Belonging (DEIB) in nursing are paramount to fostering a healthcare environment that provides equitable and compassionate care to all patients, and for each other. The 'lived experience' of the 20 nurses involved in providing narrative for this book are important, but there would have been greater depth had more of these nurses been from a black or minoritised background. DEIB is one of our greatest challenges, yet greatest opportunities in nursing, a diverse nursing workforce brings a wealth of perspectives and cultural competencies that enhance patient care by ensuring that care practices are culturally sensitive and relevant. Equity in nursing ensures that all nurses, regardless of background, have equal access to opportunities for professional growth and advancement, which promotes a more skilled and motivated workforce. Inclusion ensures that all nurses feel valued and respected, which improves job satisfaction and retention. Lastly, a sense of belonging is crucial for fostering teamwork and collaboration, which are essential for delivering high-quality patient care. Together, DEIB initiatives help create a healthcare system that is not only fair and just but also effective and responsive to the needs of a diverse patient population, this approach not only demonstrates a commitment to antiracist principles but also underscores the profession's openness to embracing multicultural opportunities.

Nursing as a profession faces a myriad of interrelated challenges that significantly impact both staff and patient care. Widespread burnout and stress among nursing staff have become endemic, driven by long hours, high patient-to-nurse ratios, and the emotional toll of constant caregiving. This persistent strain contributes to high staff turnover rates and increased absenteeism, forcing organisations to depend heavily on temporary staff who may lack continuity and familiarity with patients. The resulting instability led to historic industrial action taken by the Royal College of Nursing, who remain in dispute with the government over pay, working conditions, and safe staffing. The unrelenting pressure also causes many nurses to engage in self-neglect and emotionally log out, wherein they detach emotionally to cope with the overwhelming demands, which in turn can diminish the quality of patient care. An over-reliance on reports, inspections, and audits places additional administrative burdens on already challenged health systems, this administrative overload, combined with the aforementioned factors, leads to increased patient dissatisfaction, more frequent complaints, and ultimately poorer health outcomes. The compounded effects of these issues create a vicious cycle that erodes the morale of nurses and undermines the overall effectiveness of healthcare delivery, highlighting the urgent need for systemic reforms to support the well-being of nurses and the patients they serve.

Section two presents us with a brief vision of what the future could look like for nurses, our patients and those who lead us. I offer my own vision for nursing; a vibrant future would be characterised by a holistic transformation that addresses current challenges and embraces new opportunities for growth and innovation. This future would see the implementation of robust support systems to mitigate burnout and stress, such as more manageable workloads, increased staffing levels, comprehensive mental health support and a commitment and action to tackle racism. High staff turnover and absenteeism would be tackled through competitive pay, career development opportunities, and a positive practice environment that values and respects nurses' contributions.

In this envisioned future, dependency on temporary staff would decrease as investing in retaining and nurturing a stable, well-trained nursing workforce becomes the norm. Collaborative efforts between management and nursing staff would reduce the need for industrial action by proactively addressing concerns and fostering open communication, and nurses would receive ongoing training and support to ensure they remain engaged and motivated, preventing self-neglect and emotional log out. An over-reliance on reports, inspections, and audits would be balanced with a greater emphasis on patient-centred care and clinical autonomy. Digital advancements and streamlined administrative processes would free up more time for direct patient interaction, patient satisfaction would soar as a result of these positive changes, with fewer complaints and improved health outcomes. A culture of continuous improvement and innovation would be fostered, with nurses playing a central role in shaping healthcare practices and policies. The nursing profession would be celebrated for its critical role in healthcare, attracting new talent and ensuring a vibrant, resilient future for nursing that benefits both nurses and patients alike.

Section three introduces us to the conceptual framework of cognitive and behavioural science, the author expertly through his own experience carefully unpicks the concepts of 'overwhelm' and the impact on our lives not only as nurses, but as humans seeking to navigate a complex world. Heuristics, described in this book as 'Mental Shortcuts' play a significant role in clinical decision making, especially when quick decisions about patient care, particularly in emergency situations are time critical, the simplification of complex decision making can reduce the cognitive load required to evaluate all available information and potential options. Cognitive load in nursing, whilst not specifically discussed in the book is high in nursing, this associated with a high 'work load intensity' can have impact on the quality of care, patient safety, and well-being of nurses, thus resulting in 'mental narrowing'. Further concepts such as constraint analysis which can be used to identify, evaluate, and address limitations or restrictions that hinder our ability to perform, along with the four 'K's of knowledge: academic, skills, viewpoint and doing; these four taken together are the essential components of safe nursing and nursing leadership practice.

Fit to Care concludes with section four, the opportunity to pull together the insights from nurses, our understanding of the world that nurses practise and lead in, concepts of cognitive and behavioural science, which culminate in the Fit to Care System', a methodology based on aspirations, actions, anchors and autopilot, the importance of this system is that it puts the nurse at the centre whilst acknowledging the role they play alongside their team and the wider organisation. The opportunity to self-reflect as a nurse, to consider your 'beacon on the hill' is an opportunity seldom ever afforded during our busy working lives, the more we develop meaning in our personal and working lives, the fitter we become and the more we can achieve. Our aspirations are only limited by our ability to see beyond where we currently are, we should all have a magic wand list, ready for those moments when opportunity presents itself and we are able to advance our interests and meaning in life and at work. Anchoring our thoughts and opportunities is important, yet we are reminded that we use Anchors because both memory and motivation are unreliable, perhaps 'easification' gives us the opportunity to piggyback on already established habits that we already do on autopilot. Finally, autopilot is something we often miss out, feeling the joy of our achievements should not be underestimated, for it is this celebration that nourishes our energy and enthusiasm to continually strive for our 'beacon on the hill'. The remainder of section four connects us with our team and a helpful checklist for best practice teamwork, recognising the value of authentic care which drives a sense of belonging, which in itself brings joy to work.

Prof. Steven Hams RN, MBE, MStJ, MPH

Chief Nursing Officer

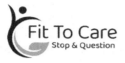

Fit To Care
Stop & Question

Want to continually improve your productivity for your stakeholders? Take the Fit to Care Insight Scorecard to identify your productivity baseline.

Discover opportunities for improvement by benchmarking your ability to capture your stakeholders' insights and the effectiveness of your meetings.

Take your free 5-minute assessment
fittocare.co.uk/scorecard

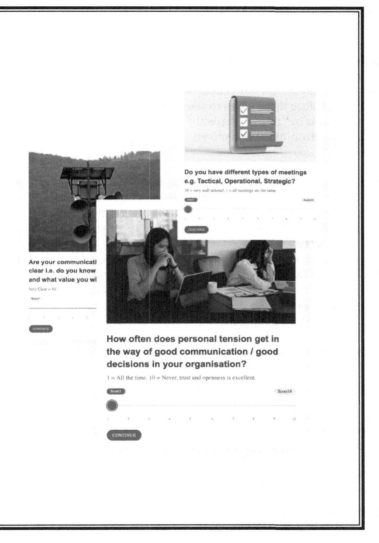

Do you have different types of meetings e.g. Tactical, Operational, Strategic?

10 = very well tailored. 1 = all meetings are the same

Are your communicati
clear i.e. do you know
and what value you wi

Very Clear = 10

How often does personal tension get in the way of good communication / good decisions in your organisation?

1 = All the time. 10 = Never, trust and openness is excellent.

Introduction

Fit To Care

Welcome to "Fit To Care". This book is not just about maintaining physical and mental health; it's about how individuals and teams can work together to provide the best possible care. It's about building stronger connections with our colleagues and improving how we serve our patients. Explore these pages to see how you can live and make your best contributions by "fitting" perfectly within your team, organisation and broader environment to positively impact the lives of every patient you encounter.

This book is for all nurses, particularly nurses in management positions who want to drive change in the NHS. I believe that nurses, utilised properly, are the backbone of the NHS, and yet currently they are underappreciated and undervalued. In an ideal healthcare scenario, nurses start their day with a well-organised shift. They are supported and empowered to seek innovative ways to enhance patient outcomes. The management team sees nurses as the "Patient's Champion" and the foundation of first-class care. Management's role is to facilitate this process. I will make the case throughout this book that such a scenario will be the secret to a sustainable and successful NHS.

I have been asked, by a Chief Nurse who I have great deal of respect, "what gives you the right to write about nurses?" It's a great question. I answered on the lines of "I have worked in and for the NHS since 2007. I have been involved in many transformation programmes and have worked closely with many nurses on my journey. I have studied what has worked and what hasn't and I have researched best practices outside the NHS too. I passionately believe that nurses and direct carers are one of the keys to breakthrough improvements for the NHS, and that is my goal – to contribute to a sustainable NHS with a happy/fulfilled workforce and satisfied patients. (Note the term patient is a generic term used throughout this book, but recognise in some settings this term is not used to describe the person receiving care from a nurse.)

The impossible can sometimes be possible.

The Beveridge Report[4], published in 1942 by Sir William Beveridge, laid the groundwork for the welfare state in post-war Britain. One of the report's ground-breaking proposals was creating a national health service that would be free at the point of use. Beveridge believed that addressing "Disease" was essential for social welfare. He recommended that the government ensure access to medical care for all citizens, regardless of their financial situation.

Aneurin Nye Bevan, the Minister of Health in the post-World War II Labour government, was crucial in implementing the Beveridge Report recommendation, leading to the establishment of the NHS in 1948.

The implementation of the NHS was so instrumental that many countries worldwide have referenced (and still do) it as a model that has influenced the development of their healthcare systems. The World Health Organization (WHO) highlighted it as a leading example of effective healthcare delivery[5].

Examples of countries that have looked to the NHS for inspiration are included in Appendix 1.

History provides the insight that just a few key people (in this case, Beveridge and Bevan), with the support of their teams around them, can be the catalyst for a fantastic revolution in Healthcare.

The NHS had many opponents and was very difficult to establish[6]. Opposition came from various quarters, including the medical profession, concerned about losing autonomy. There were also many political hurdles; the idea of a state-funded healthcare system was revolutionary and required significant legislative efforts and public support to overcome scepticism; it was an extremely tough challenge. But it WAS ACHIEVED!

This book calls for a Second Positive Healthcare Revolution, to be led by nurses, building on the foundations of the first. It will explore and make the case for the critical principles required for this revolution.

---

4 officially titled "Social Insurance and Allied Services"

5 "The World Health Report 2000 – Health Systems: Improving Performance," WHO, 2000.

6 https://academic.oup.com/ije/article/32/6/1121/775194?login=false

The 1ˢᵗ Positive Health Revolution	The 2ⁿᵈ Positive Health Revolution
(Why & What)	(How)
Universal Healthcare Coverage	To be explored
Government Responsibility for Healthcare	throughout
Free at the Point of Use	this book...

Opinions, Good Faith and "The Red Pill"

Throughout this book, I will share my opinions to help summarise each section. These opinions are based on my 16+ years of experience working for and with the NHS and references to various data analyses and insights from nurse interviews. Given the constraints of the word count of this book, some may challenge the analysis as not sufficiently comprehensive. It's always possible to do more, and I welcome challenges or additional datasets to enhance this work. Feel free to contact me for discussion and comments on my LinkedIn channel.[7]

Before we get into the details of the challenges nurses face, I hope you will consider a scene in the film, 'The Matrix', when the main character is offered to take the 'blue pill' and continue to live in blissful ignorance, or take the 'red pill' and finally see what is happening around him, even though what he sees will upset him. I implore you to take the 'red pill'. Only by opening up and revealing the actual challenges can we work together on the most appropriate solutions.

I want to make it clear that the purpose of this book is not to criticise or degrade the NHS or negatively impact the morale of the staff; quite the opposite. I aim to improve NHS morale by showing a deep understanding of the problems and by building confidence in the solutions, which will improve the lives of nurses. In this sense, it is intended as a beacon of hope.

My opinions and those of my interviewees are aired in good faith, and I believe in the interests of staff members, the wider NHS, and the general

---

7 https://www.linkedin.com/in/anthony-lawton-33617328/

public. The daily, short-term, and long-term challenges that the NHS faces are significant. However, I believe there is much that we can do to address them. This passion has driven the writing of this book.

I use references throughout to either support the data illustrated or provide additional context should the reader wish to delve deeper into a particular topic. Where there are no references, please accept these as my opinions based on my own personal experience, observations, and study.

Book Structure

This book must make a quick and efficient impact as nurses have little time. However, it must also be comprehensive, engaging, and easy to read. It is divided into five sections.

1. The first section contains real-life experiences that nurses share so that readers can understand the problems deeply.
2. The second section provides a vision of our goals from the perspectives of patients, nurses, and NHS Managers.
3. The third section focuses on cognitive and behavioural science to understand why many problems occur.
4. The fourth section offers practical systems and techniques to help fix the issues.
5. The final section provides practical implementation guidance.

The book includes many direct quotations from the contributing nurses, whose input helped to bring it to life.

The Goal & Objectives of The Book

The book aims to revitalise the NHS and nursing profession, inspiring positive changes in the lives of nurses and their colleagues. By amplifying their voices and bridging the gap with senior managers, nurses can reduce WRT (workaround and rework time), provide better patient care, improve hospital finances, job satisfaction, and career advancement. The goal is to support and develop nurses and nursing teams so they can start and end each day with a spring in their step. The key is creating an environment that allows nurses to flourish, provide excellent patient care, and ensure individual and team satisfaction.

By 2026, we aim for "Frontline First" to become the instinctive approach for public sector managers, capturing essential knowledge and experiences to enhance decision-making.

I firmly believe in the human spirit and its capacity for generosity, creativity, and kindness, especially regarding nurses. This belief is my foundation, and I will always adhere to it. My role is to support nursing managers in creating an environment that allows nurses to thrive.

The Challenges for the Nursing Profession

Nursing is a profession that has always been known for being tough. It involves delivering distressing news to patients regularly and dealing with grief every day. Young nurses must deal with significant life events with minimal professional experience, which makes the job even more complex. Additionally, extended shifts and constantly being on their feet make the job physically demanding. All these factors make nursing a more challenging profession than many jobs. When dealing with dearly loved patients, the stakes and expectations are exceptionally high.

A relevant quote from one of our 20 Nurses:

"...as a young, young girl, you know, dealing with dead bodies left, right and centre and you can't talk to anyone about it. You go home on the Tube, and you're just like, gosh, my hands have just been resuscitating a child that died an hour ago and looking around the Tube thinking none of you know that... The professional demand on your ability to cope with quite traumatic stuff is, astonishing really..."

Note that the average UK ward nurse salary is £32k[8]. The average UK salary overall is £35k[9].

 Before we discuss the more significant problems that nurses face in modern society, I would like you to take a minute to consider whether you think society currently values nurses sufficiently.

8 https://uk.talent.com/salary?job=ward+nurse#:~:text=The%20average%20ward%20nurse%20salary%20in%20the%20United%20Kingdom%20is,to%20%C2%A344%2C437%20per%20year.
9 https://www.forbes.com/uk/advisor/business/average-uk-salary-by-age/#:~:text=pay%20measures%20up.-,Earnings%20on%20the%20up,6.2%25%20compared%20to%20January%20 2023.

However, it gets even more testing! In recent times, and certainly since the COVID-19 Pandemic, there are now even more challenges:

- Intense mental and emotional strain during the COVID-19 Pandemic, which continues due to increased waiting list pressures.
- Pre-shift anxiety because of the constant and extreme pressures.
- Shifts in public attitude from appreciation to complaints about healthcare quality without considering staff shortages.
- Prevalence of negative news about hospitals and the healthcare system.
- Overwhelm and burnout.
- The stress of experiencing poor patient care (beyond nurses' control).
- Workplace dynamics and conflicts among colleagues (decreasing psychological safety).
- Gender-related challenges, political influences, and navigating diverse beliefs.
- Inadequate resources to provide the required standard of care.
- Nurses are reluctant to voice their needs due to fears of negative consequences on their positions and careers.
- The cost of living continues to impact well-being and morale.
- Community nurses feel their work is undervalued, as images of nurses on TV and in the news predominantly focus on hospital care.

The challenges nurses face are headline news, especially since the COVID-19 pandemic. Issues such as pay and benefits, staffing levels, and working conditions are all important, but the more severe impacts are on nurses' health and well-being.

The situation is worsening, with sickness rates in England on an upward trend, particularly in the North-West. In 2022, sickness absence rates were equivalent to 20,400[10] additional full-time nurses, costing the NHS around £714m[11].

---

10 https://www.nuffieldtrust.org.uk/resource/all-is-not-well-sickness-absence-in-the-nhs-in-england#:~:text=The%20reported%20sickness%20absence%20rate,4.9%25%20in%20December%202019).

11 https://www.nurses.co.uk/careers-hub/nursing-pay-guide/ With a conservative average salary for a nurse being £35,000, this loss of productivity to the NHS equates to circa £714m – on average £17m per ICB (integrated care board).

The vacancy rate in secondary care in England was 10.2% of all nursing posts, with nursing shortages impacting the medical workforce.[12] The cost of bank and agency nursing shifts is approximately £6.2 billion annually.[13]

The vacancy rates and workforce issues are particularly acute in community and primary care settings. There has been minimal growth in community nursing or midwifery, highlighting specific areas where recruitment and retention remain significant challenges.[14]

Research suggests that frontline staff in the UK are experiencing high levels of depression, anxiety, stress, burnout, and other forms of psychological distress, which the COVID-19 pandemic crisis has exacerbated. The impact on patient safety and waiting lists is irrefutable.[15]

Overall satisfaction with the NHS fell to 29% in 2022, the lowest level since the survey began in 1983[16]. The waiting list for routine hospital treatment in England could rise to more than eight million by this summer [2024], regardless of whether NHS industrial action continues.[17]

Relevant quote from our 20 Nurses:

"The nurses are on the ward with those ten patients who are deteriorating and unwell, and you can't do anything, and you have nowhere to go, and you're watching these people deteriorating before your eyes, and you can't do anything about it... the burden is a very heavy one."

---

12 https://www.bma.org.uk/advice-and-support/nhs-delivery-and-workforce/workforce/nhs-medical-staffing-data-analysis

13 https://www.nurses.co.uk/blog/stats-and-facts-uk-nursing-social-care-and-healthcare/#:~:text=There%20are%2046%2C828%20NHS%20nursing%20vacancies%20according%20to%20the%20most%20recent%20data.&text=If%20we%20add%20the%20number,a%20record%20high%20of%2011.8%25.

14 https://www.nhsemployers.org/news/latest-nhs-workforce-and-vacancy-statistics

15 Source https://www.nih.gov/

16 https://www.kingsfund.org.uk/insight-and-analysis/reports/public-satisfaction-nhs-and-social-care-2022

17 https://www.health.org.uk/news-and-comment/news/nhs-waiting-list-to-peak-at-more-than-8-million-by-summer-2024#:~:text=',- Ends&text=The%20NHS%20consistently%20met%20the,wait%20time%20is%2014.5%20weeks.

This book intends to be a beacon of hope that illuminates the path and catalyses positive change by confronting and presenting potential solutions to complex issues. Its uplifting outlook aims to inspire and empower readers to act and make a difference. We need more of this:

"I literally come home from work every day having felt I've made a big difference to people's lives. It's so rewarding. I can't tell you how much I love my job."

Nursing is rooted in love and care. I acknowledge that nurses are much more than this and I do not want to contribute to such a stereotype that can be unhelpful to the profession. As you will see throughout the book, nurses are so much more, they are professional, highly skilled and are integral/critical to the success of the NHS. We must break the old fashioned views and stereotypes, but in my view it would be a mistake to lose the power of love and care in the process. We are human and we must not lose our humanity. Improving the lives of nurses can lead to significant advancements in the NHS and, most importantly, patient care. By understanding the issues, we can make substantial improvements, ultimately benefiting us all.

The NHS, Nurses And Where I Fit In

Post-World War II, the Labour Government had the foresight to realise that a National Health Service would lift millions of people out of health poverty and, in turn, improve the well-being and productivity of the nation.

This has been held ever since (until recently, at least), and the NHS is one of the critical foundations of the UK, which was brilliantly celebrated in the 2012 Olympic games.

The chart below shows that nurses comprise a significant proportion of the NHS workforce. Given the nature of their direct care engagements, I argue that nurses are indeed the foundation of the NHS and are critically important to the whole of the United Kingdom.

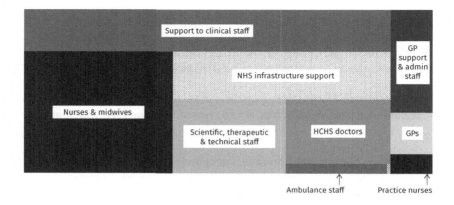

Source: Nuffield Trust analysis of NHS Digital's NHS workforce statistics, General Practice workforce statistics and Primary Care Network workforce statistics March 2022.[18]

I believe that nurses are undervalued and underappreciated.

I am not a nurse. However, I have a strong management background in health, including several years within the NHSE Behaviour Change Team, and that is why I passionately believe in transforming our current nursing crisis. My entire career and life experiences have led me to write this book and contribute to the nursing profession and society as a whole. Action has been the key to my success and will also be a prominent theme in this book.

After retiring from my career as an international showjumper, during which I represented England in 1988, my school results were terrible! However, I decided to focus on my studies and quickly excelled. I received course prizes at Sheffield University and qualified as a Management Accountant in 1999. After working in various commercial roles for Blue Chip organisations, I wanted a more fulfilling career and started working with Manchester PCT[19] in 2007. Working with the NHS changed my life forever. My Public Health innovation, "Points4Life" won Manchester PCT the National "Healthy Town" Awards and generated

18 https://www.nuffieldtrust.org.uk/resource/the-nhs-workforce-in-numbers#:~:text=Across%20NHS%20hospital%2C%20community%20and,third%20of%20the%20total%20workforce.

19 Primary Care Trust (were part of the National Health Service in England from 2001 to 2013. PCTs were largely administrative bodies, responsible for commissioning primary, community and secondary health services from providers).

a seed fund of more than £9.2m from the Department of Health, Manchester PCT and Manchester City Council.

I was a founding member of the NHS Right Care team and played a vital role in creating the "Long Term Condition Scenarios" that have been effective for CCGs since 2014. I have worked on several care pathways throughout my NHS career and deeply understand nursing and the challenges that nurses face. Recently, I served as the innovation lead for NHSE on their Menopause Optimal Pathway Toolkit for the National Programme.

"I have enjoyed working with Mr Lawton over the past three years. He has been truly amazing... His knowledge of technology blew us all away, and his hard work and dedication to our projects were second to none. He was a delight to work with and was compassionate about women's health, and I would jump at the chance to work with him again."

Janice Rymer MD FRCOG FRANZCOG FHEA, National Menopause Programme CRG Chair, Professor of Obstetrics and Gynaecology, Dean of Student Affairs, King's College London, National Specialty Advisor for Gynaeoclogy for NHSE/I.

Innovation and transformation are my areas of expertise, and nursing requires them now more than ever...

How Can This Book Assist With Such A Massive Challenge?

While the challenge is enormous, the nursing workforce possesses immense power. Working collaboratively, nursing can tackle even the most significant issues; the impossible can be made possible.

This book draws heavily on implementation experience,[20] as well as academic research in cognitive science, behaviour change, and systems thinking. The book aims to be a practical manual, avoiding complicated jargon and keeping it simple and succinct for quick and efficient use. It's designed to be action-oriented, and readers are encouraged to take notes within the book.

---

20 Particularly relevant to this book from Vervaeke / Seddon / Fogg and Lencioni. This book aims to be the catalyst for implementation within healthcare settings.

The Problems Within the NHS: Insights from Nurse Interviews

Problems Introduction

By delving into the main areas and recurring themes that have emerged from 20 recorded interviews with experienced nurses, we can better understand the deep-rooted and multifaceted causes of the problems within the NHS. We must examine the current issues more closely, as only by understanding the problems can we find the best solutions to them. This first section steers us towards a proper understanding of these issues. Sections three and four provide a comprehensive guide on why these problems persist and how we might establish practical solutions.

Research and Methodology

Twenty nurses gave in-depth semi-structured interviews over three months, from December '23 to March '24; there were many more informal conversations, including social media engagement on many of these topics. The interviews were recorded and transcribed using a tool called Otter.ai. The transcripts were loaded into a Dedoose tool to aid the qualitative thematic analysis. More than 150,000 words were captured from the nurse transcripts. The analysis process involved manually reading and "coding" significant text sections, such as sentences or paragraphs that were salient, positive, or negative. Dedoose allows you to analyse the trends and themes within these codes.

Analysis and Book Structure:

After further analysis of the interview transcripts, I found it most effective and efficient to present the data for Section 1 into four chapters, each with a specific focus. These chapters are as follows:

1. Macro Pressures – which are difficult for the NHS to influence.

2. Leadership, Management, and Culture.

3. System Consequences (impacted by 1 & 2).

4. Signals and Evidence of a Troubled System.

Under each subheading, within each chapter, I summarise the key points, provide quotes from nurse interviews to support the points, and then offer 'Key Takeaways' that we can use to develop solutions in section 4 of the book.

Chapter 1

Macro Pressures (difficult for the NHS to influence)

Macro Pressures Introduction

The NHS faces many challenges that impact its operations and service delivery. As the population ages, patients' health conditions become more complex, requiring intensive healthcare services that can strain the system. Patients increasingly have higher expectations[21] for quality and timely care, which can pressure NHS resources. (Only 24% of the public expressed satisfaction with the NHS, marking the lowest level since the survey began in 1983[22].) Political and economic constraints limit the NHS's ability to expand and innovate. Global health challenges like pandemics and international health crises require immediate responses, making routine care provision more challenging. Environmental and sustainability issues must be incorporated into healthcare planning, reflecting broader societal shifts towards greener practices. Additionally, social determinants of health highlight the need for a holistic approach to healthcare that addresses the underlying societal factors affecting health outcomes. Regulatory and compliance pressures are necessary to ensure quality and safety, but can also add complexity to healthcare delivery.

It's a demanding environment to work in!

It's common to hear in the press and on the radio how inefficient NHS managers must be and that there should be fewer managers and more nurses... **My opinion is that these views are ill-informed, and we should avoid knee-jerk reactions into thinking that NHS Management is to blame.** These factors, taken together, create an extraordinarily challenging environment for the NHS and its managers. This chapter is crucial as it examines these variables in more detail to better understand their impact on leadership, management, and the culture within the NHS, which we will explore further later in the book.

1.1   Ageing Population Dynamics

The ageing population has significantly impacted the NHS over the past two decades. With the increase in life expectancy (in the next 25 years, the number of people older than 85 will double to 2.6 million), the

---

21   https://www.bjmp.org/content/managing-patient-expectations-through-understanding-health-service-experiences

22   British Social Attitudes Survey 2023

demographic shift towards an older population has intensified, resulting in unprecedented demands on healthcare services.[23] The number of people aged 65 and over has been steadily increasing, leading to a more significant proportion of the population requiring more frequent and complex medical care. This shift affects not only the type of services required, such as an increased need for chronic disease management, geriatric care, and dementia support, but also the volume of healthcare provision needed.

Significantly, the ageing population has changed the NHS's healthcare planning and resource allocation. To cater to the multifaceted needs of older adults, the focus has shifted towards developing integrated care models. The aim is to promote ageing in place/at home and prevent hospital admissions by improving community and primary care services.

In addition, discussions have been initiated on sustainable healthcare funding, workforce planning, and technology adoption to manage the growing healthcare demands more efficiently.

> 💬 **What our network of nurses had to say on this issue:**

"... they use this online booking...it's not feasible with our elderly patients. They need that personal touch, more time, and care."

"And I think with the older nurses [more experienced] nowadays... they understand the pressures of an ageing population. But it's about getting everyone on board, adapting our practices to meet these changing needs."

"We're seeing more complex health issues than ever before... our patient demographic is older, and their care needs are more sophisticated. It's a strain on resources."

---

23 https://www.health.org.uk/sites/default/files/upload/publications/2021/InsightsReport_WEB.pdf#:~:text=URL%3A%20https%3A%2F%2Fwww.health.org.uk%2Fsites%2Fdefault%2Ffiles%2Fupload%2Fpublications%2F2021%2FInsightsReport_WEB.pdf%0AVisible%3A%200%25%20

The ageing population is putting a significant strain on the NHS, especially on nurses.[24] In an overwhelmed system, managers and decision-makers may overestimate the possible impact of software and technology and assume technology will magically solve this problem. While technology can be helpful, we must listen to the nurses; it's not a cure-all for our challenges.

By understanding the issues, we can solve them. Let there be hope!

1.2   Rising Patient Acuity Levels

The NHS is facing the challenge of rising patient acuity levels. Increasingly, patients present with more complex, multifaceted health conditions requiring a higher intensity of care, more specialised treatments, and more extended hospital stays.[25] The drivers behind this increase include the ageing population, higher prevalence of chronic diseases such as diabetes and cardiovascular diseases, and the advances in medical technology that have improved survival rates but often result in patients living with multiple long-term conditions.

Increasing patient acuity levels are having a multifaceted impact on the NHS. To manage complex health issues effectively, there is a need to shift towards more integrated care models or build on existing effective models that bring together various professionals. The trend has also highlighted the importance of continuous professional development among healthcare staff to equip them with the necessary skills to meet the challenges. Moreover, it has significant implications for healthcare planning and resource allocation, with a surge in the demand for critical care beds, specialised equipment, and healthcare workers with specialised skills.

---

24   Because nurses are the clinicians that spend most time with patients.

25   https://www.bmj.com/content/368/bmj.l6964

What our network of nurses had to say on this issue:

"We're seeing more complex cases than ever before. It's not just about managing one condition, but multiple."

"We're stretched thin as it is, and with every new technological advance, there's an expectation we can do more for our patients. It's a double-edged sword."

"The workload hasn't just increased; it's changed. We're dealing with patients who would have been in intensive care a decade ago. Now, they're on regular wards."

"When I first started, if you had a stroke, you'd be in for seven days and then go to convalescence, and now it can be 24 hours. You've got a lot more to fit in with patients who are a lot sicker or need a lot more care all of the time. Rather than having a bay of patients where two might be day five, post op where they're fairly self-caring." [The care is more intense.]

"The gender issues, the politics, the dysmorphia, neurodiversity, there's a lot more now than there ever was, and it's all added stress for nurses. Some of which are only 21 or 22 years old." [It's a lot to deal with, particularly for young nurses.]

 Key Takeaways:

Caring for patients with multiple long-term conditions while utilising new technologies in the care process exponentially increases care's complexity. Based on interviews with nurses, it is hypothesised that this complexity is poorly understood, and nurses are not fully appreciated for their role in managing such patients. Additionally, the resources and training provided to nurses are inadequate to meet the challenges posed by this level of demand.

By understanding the issues, we can solve them. Let there be hope!

1.3   Elevated Patient Expectations

Nurses have witnessed a transformative shift in how patients perceive healthcare delivery, driven by broader societal trends, technological advancements, and an increasing emphasis on patient-centred care. Patients now expect timely and effective medical treatment, a higher quality of service, greater involvement in their care decisions, and more personalised healthcare experiences.[26] This change reflects an increasingly informed and empowered patient population, with easy access to health information online and greater awareness of their healthcare options and rights.

The emergence of digital technology has significantly impacted the way patients perceive healthcare. Nowadays, patients are seeking more accessible services such as online appointments, telehealth consultations, and digital health records. Patient expectations have also risen regarding transparency and accountability in healthcare delivery, with patients demanding clear communication, respect, and dignity when interacting with healthcare professionals[27].

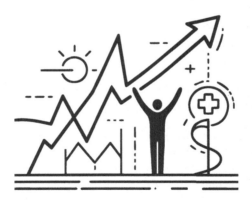

There is also an argument that higher expectations, coupled with rising waiting times within the NHS, are causing an increase in cases of violence against NHS staff.

---

26   https://ihf-fih.org/news-insights/the-impact-of-digital-transformation-on-patient-experience/

27   A recent Bain survey reveals that 65% of healthcare consumers expect a more convenient experience while 70% expect more responsiveness from providers compared with how they felt three years ago. https://www.bain.com/insights/its-time-to-elevate-the-patient-experience-in-healthcare/

The consensus among nurses in LinkedIn discussions about violence against nurses is that it is on the rise. Unfortunately, the 2023 NHS Staff Survey did not report on this due to data collection problems with iPhone users[28]. Accessing this information from individual trusts without Freedom Of Information requests is often difficult, as such data is not easily located on their websites.

If this phenomenon is related to broader societal changes (as some nurses believe), looking at the British Retail Consortium data could be insightful (given the lack of NHS Staff Survey data). In the BRC Crime Survey 2023[29], it was reported that violence and abuse against retail workers have almost doubled from pre-pandemic levels, with more than 850 incidents per day compared to more than 450 per day in the 2019/20 period.

Perhaps retail is an early indicator, and the nursing profession should brace itself for worse to come? The Royal College of Nursing offers advice,[30] including around "refusal to treat".

 What our network of nurses had to say on this issue:

"And so you were left with a set of problems to sort out, that wasn't just medical, it was the patient's expectations...they're reading things online, coming in with lists."

"We're seeing more complaints because people know what to expect, and when we don't meet that, they speak up."

"There's a clear gap between the service patients expect based on online research and what is realistically available in the NHS."

"The general attitude the whole way through the COVID-19 Pandemic was everybody thought it was great to know a nurse or we were wonderful. The minute that's finished, there's so much unpleasant stuff coming back now, where many people are complaining on every social media possible about how their care is rubbish, forgetting that there aren't many nurses left, and everyone is struggling."

---

28 https://www.england.nhs.uk/statistics/statistical-work-areas/nhs-staff-survey-in-england/

29 https://brc.org.uk/news/operations/brc-crime-survey-2023/

30 https://www.rcn.org.uk/Get-Help/RCN-advice/refusal-to-treat

"...I'm going to move you now, and they look you up on social media!" [Personal intrusion due to the patient being unhappy with being moved.]

"There is a need to provide reactive support when staff face a violent situation but more importantly, the skills to effectively de-escalate situations when they arise and to bring a heightened situation down to something manageable by the teams. Is violence on the increase? Probably. As the failures in the system increase (no ambulances to send, long waits to be seen by a GP, trolley waits in ED, delays in treatments for cancer and chronic conditions), the public is less tolerant. Therefore, anxiety rises, which, if not managed quickly, can lead to violence against our teams. We don't need 'bouncers' at every ward entrance, creating more distance between health care professionals and their patients."

 Key Takeaways:

NHS staff want to provide a first-class service, and nurses want to look after patients holistically. A new world of technology brings a whole host of new challenges and implications. Clearly, the Google factor is a material consideration, and "Google experts" can result in a lot of added pressure.

We must not underestimate the risks of increasing abuse and violence towards staff, and this needs careful attention going forward, especially if this is a growing trend, as feared by our sample of nurses.

By understanding the issues, we can solve them.
Let there be hope!

1.4   Political and Economic Constraints

Over recent years, the NHS has faced a challenging national and global environment shaped by political and economic pressures and testing public health and epidemiological events.[31] These pressures have significantly affected how healthcare is delivered, funded, and managed

---

31 Including the COVID-19 Pandemic

across the UK. Political decisions have had a significant impact on NHS funding levels, leading to austerity measures that have hugely impacted the provision of services.[32] Additionally, economic fluctuations such as the financial crisis of 2008 and other economic downturns have arguably further strained NHS budgets, leading to the need for cost-cutting measures and efficiency savings. (But everything is a choice…)

Healthcare policy in the political landscape has gone through significant changes intended to increase efficiency, reduce costs, and change the delivery of services to meet the evolving needs of our population. Certain policies have encouraged privatising some services or establishing internal markets within the NHS, sparking debates about the impact on patient care and service quality.[33]

Private hospitals in England performed more procedures on the NHS's behalf last year than ever before. The total figure of 1.67m elective (non-urgent) treatments such as joint replacements and cataract removals amounted to 10% of the total – the first time this symbolically important threshold has been reached.[34]

Brexit has also created uncertainties, particularly concerning the NHS workforce, many of whom are EU nationals, and the procurement of medical supplies.[35]

As a result, the NHS is facing severe economic constraints, which have resulted in prioritising certain services. This, in turn, has led to longer wait times for treatment and rationing of care in some areas.[36] The challenge of meeting the increasing patient demand with limited resources has led to "initiatives to improve productivity and embrace technological solutions".

---

32 https://www.bmj.com/content/384/bmj-2024-079341

33 https://en.wikipedia.org/wiki/NHS_internal_market

34 https://news.knowledia.com/GB/en/articles/the-guardian-view-on-the-privatisation-of-health-outsourcing-will-not-006e6b289413c6707922268155b2d2c866a42586

35 https://ukandeu.ac.uk/what-has-brexit-meant-for-the-nhs/

36 https://www.nuffieldtrust.org.uk/resource/rationing-in-the-nhs

What our network of nurses had to say on this issue:

"In an ideal world, you probably need double the number of staff that we have. The lack of staff is putting pressure on our ability to deliver care effectively."

"A lack of Social Care for the vulnerable elderly. Morally, that's the most challenging for all of us. Some patients in the hospital don't need to be in a hospital but there's nowhere for them to go. So we've got this bottleneck and don't have enough room in the emergency department. It's just so wrong, and it's sad to me. There were cottage hospitals when I first came into the NHS; people had their operation and went to convalesce before they went home. That's all gone."

"Oh, you can't have any more nurses. But you've got to do an extra clinic. So there's a mismatch between their expectations and putting the correct staffing on the floor to enable that to happen."

"When they remove the bursaries, you're not getting a mixture of people entering nursing. Okay. If you're a more mature student with a family, you put yourself into debt, and nursing becomes unaffordable… we're not getting the right people doing the courses."

"So we've done the business case, we've run it through, and everyone at the senior level has agreed, but there's no money. So then it turns into a waiting game. And then someone at the top will decide, knowing nothing about our service and our implications, whether or not we're allowed the money. If we're not, we still have to run the clinics and services and get told off each month because we haven't been able to do anything about it."

"Services are not safe. One of the ways to fix that would be to have legislation that says – this is the safety ratio for every ward… my analogy would be, so I fly with EasyJet. I know they aren't going to take off if there aren't enough crew on board and unless they've completed their safety checks."

"And you've got staff weeping because they can't; they're at the end of their tether. Yeah. And so I think we have to say, no, we're at capacity, no more, no more."

Key Takeaways:

During the interviews with nurses, it became evident that providing excellent care to patients is the primary goal of a nurse. University education helps to incorporate evidence-based practices into their identity. So, when the healthcare system fails to provide adequate care and contradicts best practices, it can feel like an agonising experience.

The lack of joined-up thinking across the whole care system and the removal of critical resources have colossal knock-on effects that senior budget holders do not always see or recognise.

The NHS does have access to safe staffing tools,[37] but those alone will not magically insert staff into posts; as this book explains, many issues must be tackled to fix the staff shortage.

The NHS is the foundation of a healthy UK; thus, social and political decision-makers must take funding priorities more seriously. (A recent IPSOS poll showed that 54% of Britons are prouder of the NHS than any other aspect of being British.[38]) To stress this point further from a financial perspective: "For perhaps the first time since the Industrial Revolution, health factors are acting as a serious headwind to UK economic growth. They are contributing significantly to a shrinking labour force and stalling productivity."[39]

You will see these negative effects throughout section one. Note that this does not mean the system can't be improved and made more efficient; it just shows how important it is to fund the essential infrastructure. Section four of the book will begin the journey of the solutions towards efficiency and effectiveness.

By understanding the issues, we can solve them.
Let there be hope!

---

37 https://www.england.nhs.uk/nursingmidwifery/safer-staffing-nursing-and-midwifery/safe-staffing-improvement-resources-for-specific-settings/

38 https://www.health.org.uk/news-and-comment/news/nhs-remains-our-biggest-source-of-national-pride-but-public-are-worried-about-its-future

39 Andy Haldane, former Chief Economist at the Bank of England.

1.5   Global Health Challenges

The NHS faces various global health challenges that continue to test its resilience, adaptability, and capacity to deliver healthcare services. These challenges include the rise of chronic diseases, global pandemics such as the H1N1 influenza in 2009, the unprecedented COVID-19 Pandemic that started in 2020, and the increasing threat of antimicrobial resistance. These issues have highlighted the interconnected nature of healthcare, where global trends significantly impact local health systems.

The outbreak of worldwide pandemics has emphasised the significance of global cooperation and the necessity for the NHS to be flexible in responding to health hazards that do not recognise boundaries. The COVID-19 Pandemic, for example, put enormous strain on the NHS, overwhelming its resources and requiring quick adjustments in care delivery, such as the expansion of telemedicine and the expedited deployment of vaccines.

Antimicrobial Resistance (AMR) is a complex challenge that arises due to the overuse and misuse of antibiotics. This misuse leads to the emergence of drug-resistant infections, which pose a significant global health threat. Combatting AMR requires a coordinated response, including stewardship programmes within the NHS designed to promote the responsible use of antibiotics and investment in research for new treatments.[40]

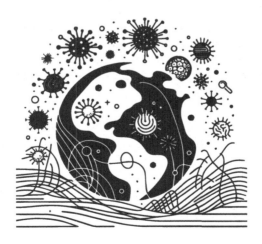

---

40   https://www.england.nhs.uk/ourwork/prevention/antimicrobial-resistance-amr/

"And so, you were left with problems to deal with, and that causes emotional strain. And this, I think, increased during the COVID-19 Pandemic because people were more alone. The teams became sporadic and worked differently."

"You were left with problems to solve on your own because everyone was trying to deal with the COVID-19 Pandemic as best as possible. It felt like we were all in survival mode, trying to keep up with the changes and ensure patient care didn't suffer."

"I also think that through COVID, everyone got moved around quite a lot, and I think that damaged things significantly. People are being trained by people who were trained in the COVID-19 Pandemic. That is not necessarily the way that you would have done it before. I know many ICU nurses have moved around so much and then burned out and were gone. They were trained for the COVID-19 Pandemic rather than for nursing in the ICU. So, I think we lost quite a lot there as well."

"Since the COVID-19 Pandemic, mental health has just gone absolutely through the roof with staff being affected by the COVID-19 Pandemic, from a personal point of view and at work. Our targets have gone through the roof because we weren't operating for two or three years. So now, for example, our waiting list was one year, but it's now two years. So, there's a push for the managers to get that back down because the government says you need to operate on people within this time. This is how long you're waiting, but no extra resources, or professionals involved in that care are on their knees."

The NHS is an incredible asset. Its resilience is only possible through the skills and, all too often, the goodwill of its staff – particularly nurses (as they are the clinicians who spend most time with patients).

Global challenges that are often unprepared for can become an enormous burden on staff, leading to burnout. The sheer scale of these challenges is just so overwhelming. We must not underestimate how significant these challenges have been and continue to be.

By understanding the issues, we can solve them.
Let there be hope!

1.6   Sustainability and Environmental Concerns

Increasingly, the NHS recognises the importance of sustainability and environmental concerns within healthcare. This growing awareness of the NHS's ecological footprint is leading to the implementation of various initiatives to reduce waste, conserve energy, and minimise carbon emissions. The NHS has become acutely aware of how environmental health impacts patient health, driving a commitment to sustainability as an operational goal and a public health imperative.[41]

Significant trends include shifting towards greener energy sources, reducing single-use plastics in medical supplies, and introducing more efficient waste management practices. The NHS has also explored the broader implications of climate change on health, recognising that the sector must adapt to and mitigate the effects of rising temperatures, extreme weather events, and the increased prevalence of diseases linked to environmental degradation.

The NHS's sustainability agenda has been formalised through strategies like the "NHS Long Term Plan" and the "Greener NHS Programme", which set ambitious targets for the organisation to become carbon neutral by 2040. These strategies encompass various activities, from

---

41   https://www.england.nhs.uk/greenernhs/wp-content/uploads/sites/51/2021/06/
B0507-how-to-produce-a-green-plan-three-year-strategy-towards-net-zero-june-2021.
pdf#:~:text=URL%3A%20https%3A%2F%2Fwww.england.nhs.uk%2Fgreenernhs%2Fwp

enhancing green spaces on healthcare properties to investing in low-emission patient and staff vehicles.

 What our network of nurses had to say on this issue:

"I was in one meeting (my mum had just died and I had a very young family), and it resulted in me telling a roomful of my colleagues to go xxxx themselves. As a mental health nurse, you know that people can break, but you don't recognise yourself. It was in a blxxxy meeting about removing my printer, and it was just the last straw." [A paper and ink saving initiative.]

 Key Takeaways:

Although every sane person recognises the importance of the environment and we MUST make radical changes, we also must understand that such a fundamental transition, in this case removing a printer, adds yet more stress and pressure to the system, which can be the final straw that breaks the camel's back, as can be seen in the above quote.

By understanding the issues, we can solve them.
Let there be hope!

1.7   Social Determinants of Health

Social determinants of health are the various conditions that impact a person's health. These conditions can include factors like the person's economic status, the level of education they have received, the neighbourhood and physical environment they live in, their employment status, and the type of social support network they have. Access to healthcare is also an important social determinant of health.[42]

The NHS has acknowledged that addressing the social determinants is critical to improving health outcomes and reducing health disparities

---

42   https://www.kff.org/racial-equity-and-health-policy/issue-brief/beyond-health-care-the-role-of-social-determinants-in-promoting-health-and-health-equity/

across the UK. They have tried to integrate this understanding into healthcare delivery, focusing on creating more holistic and patient-centred care models. This includes initiatives to improve access to healthcare for underprivileged groups, investing in community and preventive services, and collaborating with other sectors to address the underlying causes of poor health.

There has been an increasing focus on tackling Social Determinants of Health (SDH) through healthcare policies and programmes, including the Marmot Review in 2010[43]. This can also be observed in initiatives such as the Health and Social Care Act 2012[44], which aimed to enhance integration and innovation in healthcare services and public health campaigns that promote healthy lifestyles, mental well-being, and early childhood development.

The Marmot follow-up study in 2020, "Health Equity in England: The Marmot Review 10 Years On", was published to assess progress. Unfortunately, this follow-up reported that improvements in life expectancy had stalled, and health inequalities had widened since the original review. It highlighted that social conditions deeply influence the population's health and that worsening conditions over the past decade have led to poorer health outcomes. The 2020 review reiterated the need for comprehensive policies to address the vast array of social determinants impacting health, emphasising that effective action can significantly improve health across all social sections.

Commissioners invest a lot of time and energy into SDH and reducing health inequalities, as it was a significant focus in the 2019 NHS Long-term Plan.[45] However, our sample of nurse interviews reflects similar findings of the "10 years on" study...

---

43 The Marmot Review, formally known as "Fair Society, Healthy Lives," was initially published in 2010 and aimed to provide a strategic review of health inequalities in England.

44 https://www.legislation.gov.uk/ukpga/2012/7/contents/enacted

45 https://www.longtermplan.nhs.uk/publication/nhs-long-term-plan/ See page 40 Figure 13: Breakdown of the life expectancy inequality gap between the most and least deprived deciles, males, England, 2014 to 2016.

What our network of nurses had to say on this issue:

"Local authorities have faced massive budget cuts, impacting their ability to enable hospital discharges and community care. The funding for local authorities has been decimated over the last 15 years and across many different cities."

"Do we fix the road? Or do we invest in being able to pull people out of the hospital? These decisions have massive consequences for the NHS."

"We've got so much more privatised service for the care. All these care homes are private companies, and they decide what regulations or government contracts – they pick and choose. They can have beds but choose not to provide them, even when we are desperate."

"And that might be the only time that you've checked on that person's well-being if they're living alone in the community, you know, quite isolated."

 Key Takeaways:

In our society, the gap between the deprived and the privileged is widening,[46] and the NHS must play its part in health equity. This is not an option. However, we must acknowledge that this places yet another demand and pressure on the system, including the Core20PLUS5 initiative[47], and we cannot underestimate the additional strains this places on the NHS.

By understanding the issues, we can solve them.
Let there be hope!

---

46   evidence from the House of Commons Library underscores that in 2021/22, 37% of total disposable household income went to the top fifth of individuals, while only 8% went to the bottom fifth. https://commonslibrary.parliament.uk/research-briefings/cbp-7484/

47   https://www.england.nhs.uk/about/equality/equality-hub/national-healthcare-inequalities-improvement-programme/core20plus5/

1.8   Regulatory and Compliance Pressures

Over the last 20 years, the NHS has faced increasing regulatory and compliance pressures. These pressures arise from a growing demand for quality assurance, patient safety, data protection, and financial accountability within the healthcare sector. Regulatory bodies such as the Care Quality Commission (CQC) in England and evolving legislation like the Health and Social Care Act have set high standards for healthcare delivery, requiring the NHS to adapt to meet these standards.[48]

NHS provider trusts are now subject to a new Code of Governance, which took effect in April 2023 and replaced the earlier 2014 code. This new code encompasses foundation and NHS trusts and reflects broader oversight and more stringent governance practices.[49]

Moreover, the introduction of Integrated Care Systems (ICS) and the expansion of digital health technologies have increased the complexity of governance. Trusts must now manage additional responsibilities, such as system-wide collaboration involving shared planning and decision-making across various healthcare settings.[50]

The introduction of rigorous inspection regimes and performance metrics has compelled the NHS to enhance its governance structures, quality control processes, and patient care protocols. Compliance with data protection laws, especially with the advent of the General Data Protection Regulation (GDPR), has also significantly emphasised the secure handling of patient information, adding another layer of complexity to NHS operations.

Financial accountability has been another critical area of focus, with regulatory frameworks demanding greater transparency and efficiency in resource use. This has led to implementing cost-saving measures and a push towards more sustainable healthcare practices despite concerns about the impact on service delivery and staff workload.

---

48 https://nhsproviders.org/search?keywords=regulation

49 https://www.england.nhs.uk/publication/code-of-governance-for-nhs-provider-trusts/

50 https://www.mills-reeve.com/insights/blogs/health-and-care/november-2022/new-nhs-guidance-on-good-governance-and-collaborat

The intersection of these regulatory and compliance demands with clinical practice has, at times, created tensions, highlighting the balance that must be struck between administrative requirements and the provision of patient-centred care.

💬 **What our network of nurses had to say on this issue:**

"If you're working on the ward, you've got ill patients, and you're short-staffed, it's very difficult to say I'm going to the clinical governance meeting because there's no one to look after the patients. So, there's something around unrealistic expectations. Will you give up? I've given you the chance to come and talk at this meeting..." [Give up on governance because you can't leave the patients.]

"Bureaucracy, Oh, God. Yes. I mean, yeah, it's a regular thing. All you hear about is the A&E target or the fact that you've got your RTT,[51] so you become very aware of it. And you do have to fill in boxes and forms and all the rest when you've got a CQINN,[52] for example, and it's about pressure ulcers, dieticians, nutritional scores, or whatever. Then again, you've got additional rubbish to fill in."

"Feeding the beast, but you must feed the beast and feed in forms. That's where you get distracted from what you need to do."

"I would say that most matrons, in organisations, spend probably 75% of their lives in bed meetings. And that is just trying to get patients discharged. Then, you must go through a whole rigmarole to get patients discharged. You must fill in a lot of forms. You're all dragged into bed meetings because managers are keen to be seen to be discharging patients, and you could have a bed meeting every two hours. But you're forced to do so because you've got to meet your A&E target."

---

51 Referral to Treatment
52 Commissioning for quality and innovation.

Key Takeaways:

The rationale for regulation and compliance is good; it's necessary. However, when applied incorrectly and without wisdom (as we will describe later in the book), regulation and compliance can add massive pressure to the system, make the NHS unsustainable, and ultimately act against the interests of patients.

By understanding the issues, we can solve them.
Let there be hope!

1.9   Changes in Workforce

Today's young workforce has unique attitudes and expectations shaped by social media and digital technology. They seek flexibility, work-life balance, and meaningful engagement and value rapid communication, transparency, and feedback within the workplace. Social media has also made them more aware of global issues, and they expect their employers to demonstrate social responsibility and ethical practices.[53] Organisations need to adapt their cultures and policies to attract and retain this new wave of talent. It's essential to keep pace with the changing dynamics of the workforce. This isn't easy to do.

 What our network of nurses had to say on this issue:

"I used to teach sexual health when I was training at university... Tell me what you've heard... what do you think about this? What's your opinion on this? But there's no opinion, they look at you and then try to find answers on Google. Social media seems to have impacted people's ability to think and have an opinion."

"But if you go straight into nursing at 17 or 18, you're on the ward within the clinical space within a few months of starting, and you're put into very real, very difficult and emotionally taxing situations where you're going through a lot with your peers and your friends are all having a good time with no idea what's going on."

---

53   https://news.stanford.edu/2022/01/03/know-gen-z/

"When the government paid for nurses to study, what happened then was we just got people who wanted a degree that was paid for and not because they wanted to become a nurse. They thought they were coming in to do a degree like any other student, where they attend a couple of lectures a week, when, in fact, nursing courses aren't like that. Yes, you're a student in your university doing your theory, but all students are working out in practice. We don't see that as work experience. There's a good chance of getting a job in the end. So, this is how you get your hands-on training. So, you don't get paid in your course, but you get access to a job afterwards. But these students came in like any other student and then resented working for free because students in geography, history, whatever, didn't have to do that. So again, the numbers of people coming on courses are boosted, but the retention rates are terrible."

"You can teach somebody to do tasks. You can't teach somebody to be empathic, passionate, understanding, and committed – all those things that nursing needs."

 Key Takeaways:

These are brand new challenges for the NHS, and you can see that it's not as simple as "just recruit more nurses". The NHS, like many employers, needs to adapt to meet the different expectations of its younger employees.

By understanding the issues, we can solve them. Let there be hope!

Chapter 1 Summary

When I look at this long list of significant challenges, it reminds me of the Peter Kay biscuit dunking sketch. The NHS has always been very resilient, like the chocolate Hobnob, but how many dunks can it realistically take before it disintegrates like the Rich Tea biscuit – unless it adapts?

However, given the meaning, purpose, and skills that nurses (the majority of the NHS workforce) have, I believe that the NHS can change and that a Second Positive Healthcare Revolution is possible.

The challenges are tough, but there is hope, and together, the almost impossible is possible.

"Were there none who were discontented with what they have, the world would never reach anything better."
Florence Nightingale

Together for Tomorrow: Pioneering a New Era for the NHS

Chapter 2

Leadership, Management and Culture

Leadership, Management and Culture Introduction

Chapter 1 highlighted that the NHS is facing increasing levels of complexity and is under a lot of pressure. The following subheadings within this chapter will demonstrate how this pressure has influenced the NHS's management and leadership styles. Although there is a logical explanation for what's happening and why, **it's important to note that leaders and managers are not to blame.** However, for the NHS to remain sustainable, changes must be made.

2.1   Scientific Management Culture – Harming the NHS

Scientific Management's hierarchical approach can negatively affect healthcare practitioners. It can lead to demoralisation and put patients at risk.

The utilisation of Scientific Management principles[54] in the NHS has brought about a set of problematic dynamics that question the essence of healthcare delivery. This approach, which originated in the early 20th-century industrial optimisation, focuses on efficiency, standardisation, and a hierarchical division of labour. Although it appears advantageous, these principles pose challenges when applied to the intricate and nuanced healthcare environment.

The healthcare industry often focuses heavily on efficiency due to various pressures, as highlighted in Chapter 1. However, this approach can sometimes lead to a reductionist view of healthcare services. In this view, patient care processes are broken down into measurable units, which can depersonalise patient care. This means that patient needs and pursuing quantitative targets often overshadow experiences. Standardising practices – another hallmark of Scientific Management – can worsen this issue, too. It involves applying one-size-fits-all solutions to patient needs that are inherently variable, which diminishes the quality, responsiveness, and effectiveness of care.

Scientific Management's approach, which emphasises a hierarchical structure, can also negatively affect healthcare practitioners. Specifically, nurses and doctors may feel that their professional autonomy and

---

54 Scientific management principles were initially developed in manufacturing environments by Frederick Winslow Taylor in the late 19th and early 20th centuries.

judgement are stifled by the strict protocols and checklists they must follow. This can lead to demoralisation among staff and can also put patients at risk if practitioners cannot make decisions based on their expertise and the unique circumstances of each patient.

Moreover, an excessive focus on metrics and goals may divert resources and attention from essential aspects of patient care to tasks that fulfil checkboxes without contributing to outcomes.

John Vervaeke's work on cognitive science and relevance realisation[55] highlights the issues with the NHS's scientific management culture. According to his theories, complex service industries require adaptive and flexible problem-solving strategies instead of rigid adherence to predefined protocols. Arguably, the tick-box management culture enforced in the NHS impairs the staff's ability to engage in dynamic problem-solving, which is essential for dealing with the complexities of healthcare. This Scientific Management approach undermines the development of wisdom and insight among healthcare professionals, trapping them in a **cycle of procedural compliance that is not aligned with the needs of patients.**

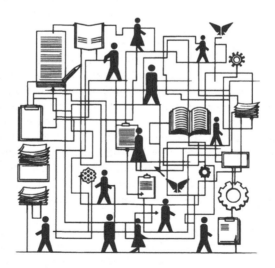

55 https://academic.oup.com/logcom/article-abstract/22/1/79/1007787?login=false

What our network of nurses had to say on this issue:

"Nursing is not medicine. Nursing is nursing care and nurturing, educating, and health-promoting. It's looking after the patient, the family, the surroundings. It's about the whole concept, and then you go into the job, and it becomes the test. When we trained, for a breathless patient, the first thing you would be thinking is, position them, give them some extra pillows, sit them up, open the window, all these basic things about looking after the person in that environment. Now, they get the doctor involved. If someone's not eating, refer them to the dietician. Well, no, if someone's not eating, check with them, check that you're giving them food they like..."

"And then suddenly you end up with a manager who is an OT[56] with no neuro background or a business manager with absolutely no nursing or clinical background. They just come in on the chief exec programme or something. I've been in meetings where someone has upset me and said, didn't you look at XYZ pathways on the web. We've been doing that for years."

"One of my ex-colleagues was visiting, and she trained me. There was a new mother, and when she got home, she was distraught because she wasn't able to breastfeed properly and was upset that the baby was distressed, too. So, my friend (helping out on Bank) did a great job and helped with the feeding and she left the woman happy and the baby was much more settled, and everything was good. She goes back and says to them, don't worry about that. I've sorted out the feeding for that lady. But she was reprimanded as 'that's not your job'."

"I think there's an issue with people having things done to them. And I think often, in a pressured environment – and most of the hospitals these days are in a pressured environment – performance, finances, and staffing have become more micromanaged."

"When I started, we were paid as student nurses, so you were much more part of the workforce. I think you were much more of a team. And there were fewer targets. Definitely fewer targets. I think there was much more freedom as well in the beginning when I first started. Yeah."

---

56 Occupational Therapist

It can be tempting to break everything down into small chunks and targets to increase efficiency in healthcare. However, this siloed approach leads to more work, more expenses, and, most importantly, a lower quality of patient care. Instead, we need to focus on seamless information flow between caregivers to provide the best possible care for the patient.

There is so much information that no one can know it all, so the information on all aspects of the patient must flow seamlessly from carer to carer. The flow is essential. This is an excellent time to recall the Socrates quote, "All that I know is that I know nothing". Our little silos are not the all-important thing. The patient is, and the "flow" of information must be seamless. For this to happen, we need to focus on communication and teamwork throughout the whole of the NHS – including Social Care. Everyone is important.

By understanding the issues, we can solve them.
Let there be hope!

2.2 "Unfitting" Targets

In a target-driven culture, there is a risk of prioritising compliance with specific metrics at the expense of the broader objective of patient well-being. This phenomenon is known as "hitting the target but missing the point".[57] In healthcare, this can lead to practices such as gaming the system, where actions are taken to meet targets on paper, even if they do not contribute to – or actively detract from – actual care quality. For example, patients may be discharged prematurely to meet hospital stay length targets, only to be readmitted shortly after, which can harm patient outcomes and increase long-term workload. (For more details, see Appendix 2, where we analyse the Mid Staff Francis Report.)

In healthcare, focusing solely on measurable targets can lead to a narrow perspective and take away attention and resources from other vital areas of care that are difficult to quantify. This can lead to

---

57   https://www.health.org.uk/sites/default/files/OnTargets.pdf The Health Foundation.

an imbalanced prioritisation, where measurable aspects of care are emphasised over more comprehensive, patient-centred approaches. This environment hinders innovation and discourages healthcare professionals from engaging in reflective practice and learning since the emphasis is on compliance rather than improvement. (Consistent with the findings within the Francis Report.[58])

Workplace stress and burnout among healthcare staff can be attributed to the pressure to meet targets (see the quotes below); nurses are rarely given explanations or rationales for collecting metrics. The high-stress environment is created due to constant monitoring and assessment and the fear of repercussions for not meeting targets. This affects the mental health and job satisfaction of healthcare workers, and leads to decreased quality and safety of patient care and a decrease in the level of compassionate care.

[···] **What our network of nurses had to say on this issue:**

"We shouldn't have to justify things in the way we are because we are doing a good job; a lot of what we do isn't quantifiable. So, it might be talking to people with cancer – with reassurance. We're providing all those skills and care that that wouldn't be provided if they cut back." [Cutbacks because not easily attributable to the "priority target".]

"I've been through several changes in the NHS; I was there when you had block contracts. If you reached your block contracts on hysterectomies, saying you've done your certain amount by September, then no one else got an operation until April. So, looking at targets that way is obviously really bad."

"And then looking at things like pathways, which can be a tick-box exercise, yeah. And don't allow individuality to come into healthcare. And you're sort of almost pushing people through a system that maybe don't want to be pushed through a system or to think about their options and stuff." [i.e. no shared decision-making.]

---

58 https://assets.publishing.service.gov.uk/media/5a7c1b11e5274a1f5cc75d16/0375_i.pdf

"There are quite a few different options. Some of them will reduce fertility, and some of them won't. You might not necessarily want to be pushed down an option that requires you to decide within four weeks because you've got to decide within four weeks. So, there are things like that. I think it's [target focus] taking away the individualised nature of the patient."

"Sometimes things are in the patient's best interest, and then you end up breaching [targets], and then you end up being fined. So, if someone's not fit for surgery and needs extra tests, the clock still ticks until they've had those tests done. But there may not be a simple quick-fix test. You can't just suspend someone (which you used to be able to do), so things can negatively impact people because you've got your targets to meet and don't want financial breaches. But also, you don't want to put someone through for an operation who's not fit."

"I've been in a meeting today where we've got to reach the four-hour ED target[59]. So, we have to change how we care for our patients to fit that target no matter what. Yeah. So, every day, even though we've got a team that works well, we're still having [to do this], I don't think you'll ever get rid of those targets."

"And I'm like, we can't; I'm not prepared for my team to move a lady whose care we haven't quite finished so that we can meet your target when that means that the care that they're going to be getting isn't as good and potentially maybe with more risk, which may then cause more problems."

"I think part of the problem has been that targets are set by somebody else, and largely completely discordant with what we are trying to achieve."

---

59 Emergency Department

Targets in healthcare aim to improve the delivery of care and outcomes. However, their implementation, often rushed and without a clear rationale, can often lead to a reductionist approach that neglects patients' complex and individual needs. This can ultimately compromise the quality and humanity of healthcare provision. We will explore this in section three of the book, but in summary, care is rarely simple enough for crude targets and tickboxes to be appropriate or relevant. Clinicians must be well-trained and have sufficient communication and autonomy to do the right things for individual patients. **Done well, performance improves without the need for dysfunctional targets.**

By understanding the issues, we can solve them.
Let there be hope!

2.3   Short Term Focus (Finance and IT)

Taking a short-term view in areas like finance and IT projects within the NHS can create numerous problems that endanger healthcare's long-term sustainability and effectiveness. Budgetary constraints, political cycles and the desire for immediate results often influence this perspective. It can lead to decisions that, while seeming cost-effective or quick in the short term, may have negative consequences.[60]

When it comes to finances, making decisions based solely on short-term goals can lead to cutting corners that don't consider the long-term benefits of investing in healthcare infrastructure, staff, and services. For example, reducing funding for preventive care programmes to meet immediate budget targets can result in higher healthcare costs in the future because of an increase in chronic conditions that require more intensive and expensive treatments. Similarly, short-term financial planning often fails to consider the growing demand for healthcare services, leading to a cycle of underinvestment that

---

60   https://publications.parliament.uk/pa/ld201617/ldselect/ldnhssus/151/151.pdf https://www.nao.org.uk/reports/nhs-financial-management-and-sustainability/ https://www.health.org.uk/topics/funding-and-sustainability#:~:text=The%20sustainability%20of%20the%20NHS,quality%20and%20productivity%20of%20care.

strains resources and compromises care quality. The pressure to deliver financial savings quickly can also lead to a piecemeal approach to funding, where investments are made in isolated projects without considering their integration into the broader healthcare ecosystem, leading to inefficiencies and inappropriate redundancies, particularly in management posts.

When implementing IT initiatives, it's essential to consider both short-term and long-term goals. Focusing solely on short-term objectives may lead to deploying technology solutions that are not in line with the NHS's strategic goals. Quick-fix IT solutions can address immediate operational issues, but they often become outdated quickly, lack scalability, or are incompatible with other systems, leading to costly replacements or upgrades. Rushing to deploy new technologies can also result in low adoption rates, staff resistance, increased risk to patients and underutilisation of potentially transformative tools due to insufficient user engagement and training. Additionally, short-term IT projects may prioritise visible technological advancements over foundational IT infrastructure and data governance practices essential for supporting integrated, patient-centred care and innovation.

Due to short-term orientations, the healthcare system constantly responds to immediate pressures instead of prioritising planning for the future. This approach leads to wasted resources and missed opportunities for improvement. It also reduces the NHS's resilience, making it less adaptable to evolving healthcare needs, technological advancements, and demographic changes. Ultimately, this short-term view detracts from the NHS's mission to deliver high-quality, sustainable healthcare by prioritising temporary solutions over comprehensive, future-focused strategies.

 What our network of nurses had to say on this issue:

"...one of our new nurse managers didn't even give me the courtesy to review the presentation. It was just like, how much money will it cost me? It shouldn't be about cost. It's about keeping your staff and keeping people healthy..."

"People are not listening because historically, that's just how things are funded."

"So, with nursing, if you prevent something from happening, it never happened. How do you tell people that that was going to happen?" [i.e. that you made a positive impact / made savings.]

"They had a meeting with the commissioner around the COVID-19 Pandemic. And instead of saying you did a really good job, you know how you have a safeguarding meeting on a virtual platform... But rather than encouraging, they just said, you didn't see enough people. We didn't get a bonus. We missed it because you didn't achieve numbers."

"The downward trend of nurse grades and support grades is due to firefighting, just to get people in. It's not an intentional strategy to downgrade. BUT then finance cuts budgets, so the original budgets for proper funding are lost. It's just short-sighted."

 Key Takeaways:

Such dysfunctions can take shape in thousands of forms, and it boils down to short-sighted silos and a lack of understanding of the patient flow and the patient's needs.

Not investing in staff might allow you to get closer to the budget this year, but the longer-term consequences for staff and patients can be catastrophic and result in many times the cost through workarounds and rework.

There is no escaping the universal truth that you must do the right things right the first time, and short-sighted, simple shortcuts always cost more in the long run.

By understanding the issues, we can solve them.
Let there be hope!

2.4 "Us vs Them" & Silos

The relentless pursuit of short-term targets and goals cultivates an "us versus them" culture within healthcare organisations, fostering divisions that undermine the collaborative spirit essential for integrated patient care.

This culture promotes isolated operations, leading to various dysfunctions. Division often arises between management, clinical staff, departments, and healthcare disciplines (primary, community, and secondary care). This negatively impacts collaborative efforts that are essential for providing integrated patient care.

Target-driven practices can contribute significantly to a divisive culture by creating competing priorities among different groups. When departments are evaluated and rewarded based on their ability to meet specific targets, it promotes a competitive rather than a cooperative mindset.[61]

Departments may unwittingly withhold information, resources, or support from one another to ensure their targets are met, which can lead to inefficiencies and a breakdown in collaboration that is crucial for the patient. NB This might not be a conscious decision; it is just a factor of focusing on siloed targets at the expense of thinking about the holistic patient pathway.

In healthcare organisations, there is often conflict between the administrative and clinical units due to the short-term focus on immediate financial and IT outcomes. Additionally, implementing new IT systems without engagement or training can frustrate the staff. They may feel that the IT department or senior management overlooks their needs and insights, pushing for rapid technological advances.

In a culture where teams work in silos, the pressure and stress can be overwhelming, resulting in a "hands-off" mentality. This means that patients are often transferred between departments without proper consideration for their ongoing care needs, with the attitude of "my job is done". This disjointed approach can disrupt the continuity of care, making patients feel neglected and other teams ill-informed.

A workplace culture that creates a divisive environment between different groups decreases the level of trust within an organisation, making it challenging to implement changes or introduce innovations. Employees may resist new ideas, feeling that they are being forced upon them by management without considering their opinions or the realities of their work. This resistance to change can impede improvement efforts, leaving the NHS unprepared to tackle the constantly evolving healthcare challenges.

---

61 https://www.bmj.com/content/363/bmj.k4907

Over time, entrenched siloes and target cultures can lead to a profound dehumanisation of the workforce and patients alike. As departments become increasingly isolated in their operational bubbles, the individuals within them start to view those in other silos not as colleagues but as mere cogs in a machine or even as impediments to their targets. This depersonalisation extends to patients, who risk being seen not as individuals with unique needs and stories but as numbers on a chart, checkboxes to be ticked, or hurdles to be cleared.

In such an environment, bias flourishes as people make decisions based on the narrow interests of their silo, often at the expense of the broader needs of patients and the organisation. The erosion of empathy and understanding can have harmful consequences, such as poor patient care and toxic workplace dynamics. Decisions made in this context are more likely to be short-sighted, misinformed, or outright harmful, which can worsen the already tough challenges the NHS faces.

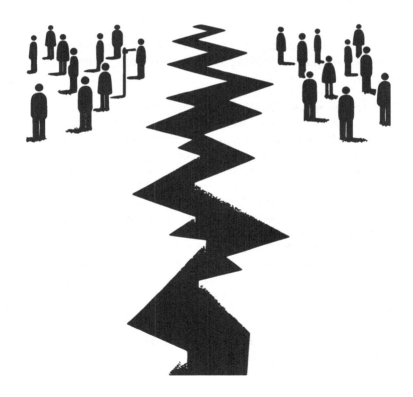

"When doctors were registrars, they'd talk to the nurses, but when they became consultants, they wouldn't have anything to do with us... they're in new groups and don't feel they can interact with the other groups."

"It was assumed that I was a nurse. I had no idea about any of the strategies. I've been patronised so many times around that. It's only really the last couple of years that I started to feel competent to talk in these places."

"Everybody who worked through that difficult time got a thank you from the directorate. They had a lovely little [gift]. And I thought that it was a really nice gesture. However, the nursing colleagues who were on the Bank didn't get one at all. So, I queried that, and I said, excuse me, I worked on this; I have worked here for decades; why haven't we got it? You're not part of our substantive team."

"The whole communication is xxxxed. No one listens to the people who know what they're talking about. No one listens to the people on the floor."

"We're in the middle of creating a new hospital. And so we've been involved. I've been involved in many meetings about this new hospital and how we can learn from our mistakes and make it to this amazing building. And so we go with our ideas, and they've got their ideas at the top, and they change everything you say to fit in with their idea of how it should work without listening, and it's been incredibly frustrating. And you think, well, some person who doesn't know how this department works is designing this hospital. We're going to have communal areas that you have to book. But that won't work if I have a sensitive meeting with a staff member. I won't have anywhere to come in and sit and shut the door and have a conversation with them. Because it needs to be this communal area because that's "the best way of working". It's not the best way of working for everything."

"Nurses aren't getting heard. They know the best way to do things, but nobody's listening to them."

Key Takeaways:

Ultimately, the divisive culture and operational silos hinder the NHS's ability to function as a cohesive, efficient entity. They detract from the organisation's primary mission of providing high-quality, holistic patient care and adapting to future healthcare needs. Here is a summary of some of the typical divisions:

Frontline Frustration: "As a nurse on the frontline, it often feels like the decisions made by management are disconnected from the day-to-day challenges we face in patient care. There's a gap in understanding what's needed on the ground."

Management's Perspective: "Balancing the budget and meeting clinical needs is a tightrope walk in healthcare management. It's challenging to allocate resources to satisfy all parties, including frontline staff."

Resource Allocation Conflict: "We're constantly pressured to do more with less. It seems the management doesn't realise how resource constraints directly impact patient care."

Communication Breakdown: "There's a real need for better communication between management and clinical staff. Without open dialogue, misunderstandings and a sense of division only grow."

Policy vs Practice: "Policies formulated at the administrative level often don't translate well into practical, bedside patient care, leading to frustration among healthcare professionals."

Various instances show that narrow, self-centred objectives precede a collaborative approach prioritising the patient's well-being. We need to foster a more robust culture of teamwork and collaboration.

By understanding the issues, we can solve them.
Let there be hope!

2.5   The Perils of Over-Siloed, Over-Simplified Systems

The NHS has a paradoxical problem with its team structures. While breaking down tasks into smaller units may make them appear more straightforward and manageable, it introduces communication barriers that lead to inefficiencies and errors. This fragmentation results in excessive handover events, causing potential loss of critical information, misinterpretation, and delays. This can ultimately lead to adverse patient outcomes such as longer wait times, repetitive assessments, and a higher risk of misdiagnosis due to the lack of holistic care.

Rather than streamlining operations, the silo mentality inflates bureaucracy and operational waste, which significantly undermines the efficiency of the healthcare system. Ironically, the NHS's attempt to simplify tasks by compartmentalising functions leads to a more convoluted, less patient-centric, and ultimately less effective healthcare system.

John Vervaeke's chessboard analogy illustrates the concept of combinatory explosion. This explains that the number of potential legal moves in chess exceeds the number of particles in the universe. It is a powerful metaphor for understanding the complexity of the NHS (which has far more variables and rules than chess). Just as a chess player navigates this vast number of possibilities through strategy, intuition, and experience, managing the NHS requires a similar, if not more profound, depth of wisdom. The NHS, with its vast web of services, stakeholders, and patient needs, presents a complexity that dwarfs the permutations of a game of chess. This complexity cannot be managed by rigid protocols or hierarchical decision-making. Such governance creates an illusion that we know what we are doing and have all the answers – but we don't. We're just making things even more complicated! "Simple" decisions or rules often fail to foresee the dysfunctional consequences.

"And that's another problem: There isn't always a career pathway unless you want to go into management. You're stuck at a certain level. Yeah. And so that's why people don't want to go into that area. Yes, there isn't any progression, and a lot of the posts have been changed, and a lot of the banding has been downgraded. And so, you lose experience through that as well." [We are not developing wisdom within the system. Rules about progression become dysfunctional.]

"You might find (like with MS nurses) that somebody in charge of a team might be band 8 in one place and band 6 in another, which is quite a large difference in money." [Silos resulting in inconsistencies and unfairness.]

"So, the highest people hierarchically in medicine and consultants still see patients operating; they still see them in outpatients and are still doing ward rounds. But that isn't true of nursing, and that's really different. So, the most senior nurses, and I'm thinking about nursing leadership, across the NHS, are not in the clinic; they might come around and visit. So, the way the nursing system is set up is that your value becomes higher and higher the farther away you become from patient care. It's the same in primary care, too." [The argument here is that this nursing systematic approach to removing senior nurses from the direct care is not helpful and creates more silos.]

"Some organisations will not let a band 6/7 go part-time and stay on their same grade, especially when nurses are semi-retired, as they are expected to take a lower grade and salary." [Different rules for different silos.]

"So, in primary care, we do have locum nurses. The difficulty with using locum staff is that they don't pick up the admin generated by that session. It's the same with a GP, who can come in and do a clinic but not clinical admin. So, the blood tests that were ordered need somebody to read the results. Who's that person? It's not great for patient continuity."

Vervaeke's insight into the necessity of wisdom underscores the importance of harnessing collective skills, experiences, and perspectives within the NHS. In this context, wisdom transcends mere knowledge; it involves the integration of diverse insights, the capacity for judgment, and the flexibility to manage unforeseen challenges.

Therefore, the effective management of the NHS hinges on an approach that values and synthesises the contributions of all its members, from frontline staff to senior administrators. By fostering a culture that embraces this multiplicity of perspectives, the NHS can cultivate the wisdom required to navigate its complexities, ensuring a more responsive, resilient healthcare system that is more attuned to the holistic needs of those it serves. We will address how to do this in Section 4.

By understanding the issues, we can solve them.
Let there be hope!

2.6   Lack of Wisdom:

The lack of "wisdom"[62] in the NHS manifests itself through undervaluing its staff members. By failing to recognise the intrinsic value of healthcare professionals, not listening to their insights, and restricting their autonomy, the system squanders the skills and perspectives they offer and impoverishes itself. This lack of wisdom is not a mere oversight but a systemic flaw that diminishes the potential for excellence and innovation within healthcare delivery.

Staff dissatisfaction is a direct consequence of this oversight. When healthcare professionals feel undervalued, their motivation drops, their commitment falls, and their capacity for empathy and innovation is reduced. The wealth of experience and insight that could be harnessed to improve patient care and foster a more collaborative environment remains untapped. This exclusion leads to a workforce that feels alienated and a system that operates well below its potential.

---

62   The context of this will be explained later in section three of the book.

The implications of this disregard extend beyond staff morale. Patients suffer the most. In a system where staff are not listened to and where their autonomy is curtailed, the quality of patient care inevitably declines. For nurses and other healthcare professionals who enter the field with a passion for caring and a commitment to patient welfare, witnessing poor patient care is profoundly distressing. The dissonance between their professional values and the realities of a system that fails to capitalise on the wisdom within its ranks can lead to burnout and an increased sense of helplessness.

> 💬 **What our network of nurses had to say on this issue:**

"Because of the demands on the service, people aren't going to train in things. So, I know MS nurses who have been newly put in posts that have never done any work in MS before, who have not been allowed time off to go to their training, and so when talking to patients, they don't know what they're talking about. Because their managers won't give them the time off to do the training to get those skills under their belt, which has a massive impact on patients."
[Wisdom is not part of the culture.]

"...thinks that nurses are just here to empty bedpans. People don't treat people as well as they should because they don't feel that their role is important." [Every role is very important as all things are connected.]

"It's that short vision that the NHS often has: Let's not look at the real problems. Let's just put a plaster over things. Yeah, you haven't dealt with the actual wound itself." [A lack of wisdom impacts on the quality of decision making.]

"I think part of the issue within nursing is that nurses get promoted to management positions without any management training. And you must have nurses managing nurses, but they also would benefit from much stronger HR support. They're getting a load of grief because whatever's happening, targets aren't being met. They don't quite know how to get the best out of their staff. So, they try to tell them off and tell them they've got to do this rather than listening to them and saying, well, how can we make this better?"

"We have very good knowledge and expertise in managing people and spotting situations that others will completely miss. We also

*know what's going wrong and how to get better." [The knowledge
and wisdom is there; it needs to be shared and utilised.]*

*"The person that used to manage me would never have seen me
work. Never saw how I worked in clinic. I think people are very
much tied up with the management of targets, risks, and complaints
and go into meeting after meeting after meeting without any time
to physically go to places or be somewhere, so I think there is a
disconnect there."*

Key Takeaways:

Ultimately, the lack of wisdom in valuing and engaging with
the NHS staff not only impoverishes the system but also erodes
the foundation of quality patient care. It underscores a critical
need for a paradigm shift towards a management approach
that recognises the invaluable contributions of every staff
member, fosters their development, and leverages their diverse
perspectives for the collective good. We must move upstream
and prevent the risks and complaints before they develop. Only
through such wisdom can the NHS overcome its challenges
and fulfil its mission of providing compassionate and effective
healthcare.

**By understanding the issues, we can solve them.
Let there be hope!**

2.7   Stagnant Learning, Development, and Strategic Career Pathways

The NHS has a significant issue that stems from focusing too much on
tasks and targets rather than the overall well-being of its staff. This
approach overlooks the essential elements of personal growth, learning,
and career progression necessary for a thriving healthcare environment.
When measurable outputs and short-term goals are prioritised, the NHS
struggles to adapt, innovate, and provide high-quality care.

**In a culture that values productivity and meeting targets, investing
in continuous learning and development is often seen as a luxury**

rather than a necessity. Unfortunately, this perspective leads to limited opportunities for skill enhancement, career growth, and role evolution. Staff members may be stuck in a cycle of mundane tasks, with little chance for professional development or exploring new roles and responsibilities. This not only hinders personal fulfilment and job satisfaction but also deprives the healthcare system of the diverse skills and perspectives needed to tackle the complex challenges of modern healthcare.

The absence of focused career paths in healthcare can lead to dissatisfaction. Employees without clear personal and professional growth direction may become disengaged and less committed to the organisation. This can result in higher turnover rates and valuable experience and knowledge loss. This scenario can be particularly harmful in a field where skills and roles continually evolve to keep pace with medical science and changing patient needs.

As you can see below, the dysfunctions of not understanding and managing roles well are also detrimental to the service and all involved.

> 💬 **What our network of nurses had to say on this issue:**

"In the wider context there are too many instances of getting people to do roles that they're not trained or competent for. And then wondering why something like reassessments are not done and then wondering why operations are cancelled. It's because you've just told the band 5 to do pre-assessment, but not explained the importance of what goes behind it."

"And so, we're struggling to recruit people into specialist nursing roles because you might be worse off in terms of money than you were before because you're not getting the enhancements or night shift increases."

"Nurses are not very good at saying what they do, so somebody else will come out and take that ground, like a clinical specialist. So, physios and OTs are coming, but they might not be able to do the medication management or manage it, but they also bring different things to the mix. But it's also about protecting the nursing role because I feel that's been going away over the last few years."

"And also, in large organisations, there are these unwritten rules, and people sometimes don't want to train new people because they feel like they're taking their places. So, there's been articles about nurses eating their own, that sort of thing. So yeah, people keep things to themselves..."

"New roles suddenly came out, but there was no conversational communication around what you think works. So I guess I don't feel part of any development."

"The computer says no, mentality. It seems that all this technology we've got from a nursing perspective, we've become more medical than nursing, holistic, caring for the person... when my dad was in there, I said, he's fractured six ribs, and he's only had one paracetamol. And to my disbelief, the nurse said, no, it's not been four hours yet."

"There's no consistent structure around changes within your role and boundaries. There's no structure to mentoring."

"The ability for nurses to progress in their careers has massively been impacted by the fact that we're now training nurses to do Doctor jobs, which is ultimately what we're doing."

"We've now got university-based education that is very much focused on pre-registration nursing. Some of the post-registration stuff is geared towards things like advanced clinical practice, which is fully under the umbrella of medicine and not under the umbrella of nursing. We're decimating the nursing hierarchy and structure as we advance."

 Key Takeaways:

Ultimately, by neglecting the importance of learning, development, and strategic career planning in pursuing narrow targets, the NHS risks compromising the morale and satisfaction of its workforce and the quality of patient care.

By understanding the issues, we can solve them.
Let there be hope!

2.8   Staff Care, Supervision, and Lack of Value

Nursing is a tough job that demands a lot from those who choose it as a profession. It's not just about dealing with the technical and intellectual challenges, but also about the emotional and physical burden of caring for others. To help nurses cope with these demands, they must have dedicated time for supervision and care beyond their professional learning and development.[63]

Women also have several unique challenges. The menopause is an example of a crucial phase in the lives of many nurses, along with having children, and women often bear the brunt of bereavements (women frequently take on substantial emotional labour during bereavement, navigating both their grief and facilitating the grieving process for others around them[64]). Recognising and addressing these unique challenges is essential for promoting well-being and sustaining the workforce. Providing comprehensive support and understanding within the healthcare environment is crucial as nurses undergo this significant life transition. By doing so, we respect their invaluable contribution and ensure that the nursing profession remains strong, resilient, and responsive.

Supervision in nursing is more than just oversight or managerial control. It's about creating a supportive framework where nurses can reflect on their practice, discuss emotional burdens, and seek guidance on complex cases. Providing this kind of support is essential in preventing burnout, a common issue in the profession. By allowing nurses to share their experiences and challenges openly, supervision acts as a valuable outlet for the stress and pressure of the job.

In addition, offering dedicated care for staff, including mental health support, physical wellness programmes, and initiatives to encourage a healthy work-life balance, is crucial for maintaining a resilient nursing workforce. Recognising that nurses are human beings with personal needs and addressing those needs holistically is vital in sustaining their motivation and commitment. Investing in staff well-being enhances

---

63 https://www.nursingworld.org/~4aaf68/contentassets/
ce8e88bd395b4aa38a3ccb583733d6a3/understanding-and-prioritizing-nurses-mental-health-and-well-being.pdf

64 https://together.stjude.org/en-us/for-families/bereavement/gender-differences-in-grieving.html

job satisfaction and directly translates to improved patient care. When nurses feel cared for and supported, they are better equipped to provide compassionate, high-quality care to their patients.

However, the opposite also applies. When they don't have a supportive framework, staff can soon feel isolated, stressed and less able or even unable to do their jobs. System pressure and "Us vs Them" cultures can exacerbate these problems, even to the point of racism being far more prominent than most of us would expect; i.e. the culture becomes tribal and confrontational rather than united with a focus on the patient.

 What our network of nurses had to say on this issue:

"As a young girl, you know, dealing with dead bodies left, right and centre, and you can't talk to anyone about it. You know, you go home on the Tube, and you're like, gosh, my hands have just been resuscitating a child that died in my hands an hour ago and looking around the Tube thinking none of you know that... and you don't have any debrief or ability to say that you're struggling with any of that, then you're considered just not pulling your weight or not cut for the job sort of thing."

"I think people don't feel supported, essentially, yeah. And they don't feel heard."

"For example, our nurse consultant recently retired, and they temporarily replaced her with a locum Doctor consultant whose pay is significant. She worked in our clinics alongside my colleague X, a band 8, who's on half the salary. She was asking for help, which is fine, you know, but then you have to recognise all staff as well."

"If you answer emails or do something, sometimes it comes back to bite you because then you get more emails and get bombarded. Yeah, the person next to you gets nothing because they didn't answer them for six months."

"It's fair to say you're not being respected for the work you're doing for the role you're doing."

"It's really interesting. It's very different in Australia. They are seen as professionals and as qualified professionals. It's respected. The salary

*is better, and potential career levels are higher, but it's just that the
perception from patients and others is quite different. Whereas in
the UK, there is this still quite patronising attitude, and that's what's
coming out recently on social networks."*

*"They don't like to be in an environment where they constantly feel
scared; they feel that people are not going to support them if there is
an issue or an incident."*

*"We wanted to sort out, have a coffee room, a nice quiet area, etc. We
got together, and a parent who knew somebody who's a painter and
decorator came in and completely decorated the staff room for us. It
was much more relaxing because we had a dirty, smelly hole before.
So, it makes them feel a bit better, and our team now sees that things
are beginning to get done. But if you want them done, you've got to
do them yourself."*

 Key Takeaways:

In an environment as complex and fast-paced as the NHS, where
the demands on nursing staff are equally as complex and fast-
paced, ensuring that nurses have access to robust supervision and
comprehensive care is not just important – it's essential. Every staff
member must be treated with respect and seen as a critical part of
the jigsaw so that they can focus on the patient. It's then possible
to break the barriers, break the silos, and break the "Us vs Them"
dysfunctions. The patient must become the common denominator,
the consistent belief for all.

***By understanding the issues, we can solve them.
Let there be hope!***

2.9   Over-reliance on Regulation and Compliance (lack of trust)

A further challenge faced by the NHS is excessive focus on following
rules and regulations and, therefore, substantially less reliance on
professional judgment and autonomy. This approach has resulted in a
culture of fear and defensiveness among healthcare staff, who are more
concerned with compliance than exploring innovative solutions for

patient care and have little time for the latter. Compliance requirements can drain morale and detract from patient interaction and care planning, which is far from ideal.

The emphasis on rules and regulations often leads to a one-size-fits-all approach, ignoring unique patient needs and circumstances. This can result in suboptimal patient outcomes as the flexibility to tailor care to individual needs is lost. The lack of trust implicit in this system undermines the professional autonomy of healthcare workers, particularly nurses, who are trained to make nuanced judgments about patient care.

Over-reliance on compliance mechanisms can also create a blame culture and inhibit open communication within the NHS. Staff may be reluctant to report errors or near misses for fear of punitive responses, thereby missing crucial opportunities for learning and improvement. Instead of fostering a culture of continuous learning and safety, the preoccupation with regulation and compliance can perpetuate a blame culture, further entrenching the lack of trust and stifling the collaborative spirit necessary for high-quality healthcare delivery.

Compliance and governance are crucial in healthcare to ensure patient safety, maintain high standards of care, and uphold ethical practices. However, it is essential to strike a balance that respects these protocols without stifling professional judgment and innovation with a rigid "computer says no" mentality.

 What our network of nurses had to say on this issue:

"This morning, I've been writing a business plan for a third nurse in our team, and there are so many hoops to go through. It's stress. So much time, and it's taken me away from patients… but they don't see the value. Very rarely will the NHS give you another Parkinson's nurse. Yes, I think it's interesting that we have to go through this dance every time, even though the value of specialist nurses is huge."

"I suppose in some ways, much more stuff is regulated. A lot more stuff is defined by your role and your grade. And that can hold people back because people don't want to be seen as going outside of their role. And this is what I do as a band x, etc. Whereas I think

when I first started, we were quite willing to do different things for experience and try and get on and it was different banding anyway, so I think Agenda for Change has definitely changed things."

"The onus for everything regarding performance is on the manager, so you have to put a plan in place for anyone not performing to improve. You give them step one, step two, etc. And then, if they're still not developing at that point, then theoretically, you could dismiss them, but that never, ever happens."

"They are very driven by guidelines and protocols, and they don't actually think outside the box, whereas I think there should be a bit more critical thinking and autonomy."

"We get so hung up with getting it wrong that we can't get it right."
[In the context of struggling to work with patient data across different organisations.]

"And I think with the older nurses nowadays, we have seen things go around in circles. They'll put one policy, then change it, and then they'll put another policy, which goes round in circles. But this time, it feels different. I think, and I think a lot of people have said it this time. It does feel like a crash point when it comes to the NHS."

 Key Takeaways:

When it comes to healthcare, compliance is essential for safe practice. However, it's equally important to avoid a rigid approach that hinders professional judgment and innovation. In interviews with nurses, they shared that a culture which values healthcare professionals' expertise and wisdom is essential. By fostering such a culture, compliance can be a foundation for safe practice rather than a barrier to adaptive and patient-centred care.

By understanding the issues, we can solve them.
Let there be hope!

Chapter 2 Summary

Chapter 2 illuminates the complexities of managing the NHS, which are often overlooked. Some argue that investing more in management structures is necessary because the NHS is known for its lower management spending than other international health systems.[65] However, I believe that our initial focus should be on addressing the issues raised in this chapter. We need to break down barriers, improve the culture, and prioritise the needs of patients. By listening to our nurses (as Patient Champions), and putting patients first, we can start the process of transforming the problems within the NHS and making the NHS sustainable again.

---

65 https://www.nhsconfed.org/articles/are-there-too-many-nhs-managers#:~:text=The%20 NHS%20is%20under,3%20per%20cent%20in%202023)%20.

The challenges are tough, but there is hope and together the almost impossible is possible.

"How very little can be done under the spirit of fear" **Florence Nightingale**

Together for Tomorrow: Pioneering a New Era for the NHS

System Consequences (from Chapters 1 and 2)

System Consequences Introduction

In the previous chapters, we examined issues impacting the NHS, such as the pressure it faces, its management philosophy, and its targets. In this chapter, we will focus on the specific effects of these problems on the NHS's efficiency, the well-being of its staff, and the quality of care it provides to patients.

3.1   Increased Workload (Workaround and Rework).

Workarounds and Rework arise when a service fails to do something right the first time for the patient, leading to additional work in the system to correct the initial error. This concept is pivotal in understanding the inefficiencies and unnecessary workloads that trouble the NHS.

This additional work represents a significant waste of resources, as time and effort are diverted from value-adding activities to address preventable errors and oversights. This resource misallocation is inefficient and costly, detracting from the NHS's capacity to improve and innovate.

Temporary solutions known as workarounds may seem innovative, but they are often a sign of deeper system problems. These quick fixes involve healthcare professionals bypassing procedural bottlenecks (often unknowingly), which can show adaptability but also highlight the system's inefficiencies. While seemingly necessary and often appearing to produce the desired outcome, these ad hoc solutions perpetuate the root cause problems and continue the inefficient workaround and rework. This adds to the overall workload and stress, which increases the risk of errors and inconsistencies.

Healthcare staff face significant burdens due to extra work caused by workarounds and rework. This leads to burnout and low job satisfaction, taking time and resources away from patient care.

> 💬 **What our network of nurses had to say on this issue:**

"At the moment, we're going through a transformation at work. It's an organisational change that they want to change how things are run, but they haven't thought about how patients come into the

system. It's like, you need to discharge them because we're worried about the safety risk... If you discharge them and lose the follow-up, it's not until they end up in A&E that you've got a whole load of new problems to deal with, which takes twice as long."

"I used to dictate discharge letters, and they used to be sent to somebody somewhere else, who then sent them on somewhere else. You got them back eventually, and you're looking, for goodness sake, they've interpreted it completely wrong, and it doesn't make sense. And so, in the end, I just thought this was ridiculous, and you should address the problem. I know, but sometimes it's quicker to do it yourself, which is wrong."

"I'll be back in a minute, is a very common problem because you then set patient expectations and also, I think, phoning people back. When you ring someone back, they're surprised you've rung them back because they're used to just having to ring and ring and try to find someone to speak to." [Patient workarounds and rework.]

"We're not relying [on GPs] that we could leave to them to do it. We are holding on to patients, I think because we're a bit anxious about things..." [Concerned about the functionality of Primary Care at the moment.]

"So, I think that there's a certain sort of blinkers on, and I'm just going to get through what I've got to because it's too much. Yeah, not answering call bells because there's not enough staff, which is really difficult." [Ignoring things doesn't fix them.]

"If we had somebody just to take all of those calls, answer an inbox, triage, all of those things that don't need a clinical, expert opinion on, and then anything that is going to be easy, it could be triaged or diverted towards us. That probably takes up much more time than it should, and it takes us away from patient contact. It's poor management of clinics, poor booking systems and patients being booked into the wrong clinics. Poor management of operating lists takes a lot of our time as specialists and nurses away from patients and questions of appointments being booked incorrectly."

"There's a huge demand for appointments and great big waiting times, so this patient complains that there were issues with appointments. Instead of the managers trying to book the appointment, they are too *busy, so they don't answer their emails, and they don't get to it, and the appointments aren't made even though they should have been made. So, then the patient gets crosser. Then it comes through as a complaint that gets managed by three managers who then bring it back round, then give it to [very senior clinician] and say, could you please find an appointment for this patient who's complained? So, it's like three sets of management time because one person didn't answer the email at the first point to book the appointment. So, it just makes a whole load more work. Because at the ground level, there isn't enough staff to do the basic work that needs to be done."*

"A prime example was my dad; he's been very independent but had a bad fall recently and ended up in the hospital. I think we'll need to change the bed; he's been incontinent. But my dad is not incontinent. So instead of working out why he wasn't getting to the toilet on time because he was in pain and worried about falling, so he didn't want to go, they stuck a pad on, and that was the answer! There was no forethought. He'd been on powerful analgesia, and then nobody checked that he might be constipated; it wasn't proactive care at all, which then creates problems down the line."

 Key Takeaways:

The NHS needs a "Systems Thinking" overhaul to improve patient care and reduce unnecessary workloads. The root causes of Workarounds and Rework are poor communication across silos (teams and departments), and a lack of emphasis on getting things right the first time, FROM THE PATIENTS' PERSPECTIVE.

Nurses must feel they are working within a culture that values learning, curiosity and continuous improvement. This will result in much more "right first time" work.

The initial reset will require some extra resources so people can step back and see all the waste. But when systems are improved, much work will dissipate, pressure will be reduced, and patient care will improve.

By understanding the issues, we can solve them.
Let there be hope!

3.2　Overwhelm, Burnout and Decreased Morale Among Staff

Healthcare professionals face a significant challenge known as "Workaround and Rework", as seen in 3.1 above. It generates extra work and makes their job less efficient. By creating more tasks through errors and corrections, staff members must deal with more work than necessary. They need to care for patients physically while managing administrative work like correcting mistakes, documenting issues, and dealing with rework processes. This extra workload can be overwhelming and affect the overall well-being of healthcare professionals and the efficiency of the healthcare system.

The high workload in healthcare has significant effects on staff. Firstly, the number of tasks can lead to physical exhaustion since healthcare professionals work longer hours, under intense pressure, to manage their regular duties and additional demands. The emotional toll is significant. Dealing with preventable errors and knowing that these issues negatively impact patient care can lead to feelings of disillusionment and professional inadequacy. This was comprehensively exemplified during the COVID-19 Pandemic when the use of PPE in line with infection prevention and control added multiple layers of stress, such as time taken donning and doffing PPE, communication difficulties between all parties due to wearing of masks, limited contact with patients such as hand holding, and complex decision making.

When healthcare professionals are continuously overloaded with work, it often leads to burnout – a state of exhaustion that affects the mind, body, and emotions. Burnout affects the health and happiness of healthcare professionals and their ability to provide attentive care to patients. This creates a cycle of Workaround and Rework demand, increased workload, and burnout that harms staff morale, leads to more absenteeism and turnover, and challenges the sustainability of the healthcare system; it's a vicious cycle.

 What our network of nurses had to say on this issue:

"I'm rarely out before 10 in the evening, 14-hour shifts. They said oh, if you had a chance to have lunch, what's lunch? It's been sitting in the fridge all day, and I'd take it at 10 pm. And you think this is absolutely nuts, and I know you should make time to have lunch, but

as soon as you sit down, the crash beep's going to go, or you know that something else will pop up... there's so much pressure."

"Some people get the Sunday scaries, you know, in a job because when you're working shift, but this could be any day of the week, and I would start to feel the anxiety creeping in. I mean, half the day before, and it would impact how I was going about my days or feeling. You'll be at your friend's, and you'll think I've got to work 13 hours, and you have no idea what will happen."

"The stressful things are not having enough nurses, not having enough time, and then you end up not being able to take a break, not being able to have anything to eat, not being able to go to the loo. I mean, it's a running joke, but a nurse's bladder, I can go a whole day without going. And then you think, how am I going to be able to get off on time? You never make plans and must be up early, so you don't sleep well. And then you're worrying about who will be in the next day."

"There are two of us, and we have a caseload of 700 patients. So, there must be transparency with the patients. We are there for them; we don't want to disappoint them, but there will be a time limit to when we can get back to them."

"It is getting to be unsustainable, and the system is broken. And the system is there because of people like me and my colleagues who work overtime, give ridiculous amounts of goodwill, and bind together. And I've been in very toxic teams."

 Key Takeaways:

Human beings can only take so much; everyone has a tipping point. Addressing the root causes of Workarounds and Rework (systems thinking with a focus on the patient) and reducing unnecessary workload is essential to safeguarding the well-being of NHS staff and critical for the NHS's sustainability.

By understanding the issues, we can solve them.
Let there be hope!

3.3   Blame and Psychological Safety[66]

When workloads increase, people can quickly burn out and are much more likely to make mistakes. This can lead to increased pressure, guilt, and a culture of placing blame, which can cause a lack of safety for people to speak up and work together effectively. When this happens, it can negatively impact teamwork, innovation, and patient care.

In a workplace where blame is the norm, staff members may worry about facing consequences for their mistakes. This fear can make it hard for them to report errors, close calls, or to speak up about their concerns. This lack of communication and transparency is a big problem for any organisation that wants to learn and grow. Without a feeling of safety, healthcare professionals are less likely to reflect on their work, share what they know, or suggest new ideas. They're afraid of being judged or punished. This kind of environment will hurt their professional development and limit their ability to identify and fix more systemic problems. This can lead to inefficiencies and care gaps that will persist over time.

When team members can't feel safe expressing themselves, their trust in each other and team cohesion can be undermined. This can lead to poor collaboration as individuals become less willing to work closely with others, become more guarded, and are much less likely to share their errors or near misses. These issues can negatively affect patient outcomes, which can cause disjointed care delivery due to a lack of coordination and mutual support.

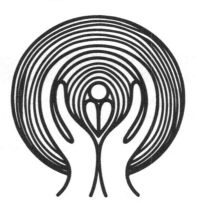

---

66 Harvard Business School professor Amy Edmondson, first coined the phrase "team psychological safety"

What our network of nurses had to say on this issue:

"I was called at three in the morning by a healthcare assistant because the nurse on duty was standing in the waiting room of our walk-in emergency unit, having a screaming row with the on-call doctor. You know, throwing racial slurs at each other, it's three o'clock, and I was like, I don't know what to do. They're just screaming at each other in the waiting room with patients there."

"The students see a completely different way of doing things from how we've told them. We're telling them to challenge, but because the stress level in practice is so high, they don't because they need someone to sign off on their record. So, they won't cause any conflict because that will reflect badly on them. And it just ends up with a lot of dissatisfied people."

"They are very afraid to speak out and criticise anything. Also, they think their jobs are on the line. Yeah. And I don't know that that's changed dramatically. I think towards the end [retirement], when I knew I was going, I felt a lot freer. You didn't have to rely financially on the job."

"When we come to say what we need, we don't just go to that because we're worried. Historically, we never stood above the parapet to say what we were doing because you'd likely lose your posting if you did that."

"And then we'd beat them up because they do it wrong. And then they get disillusioned and think, why should I bother doing all this for this amount of money because all you do is moan about it?"

"But then when you're slapped down on high despite highlighting all the potential risks and the lack of continuity or the fact that these patients aren't going to be receiving the care, it's quite frustrating and a little bit soul destroying, but yeah, I continue to do it because it's really important."

"There's a blame culture, which stresses nurses out, especially if something happens. So, if that could be changed somehow, I would consider returning to the NHS in the future, but what probably frightens me the most is that this big beast doesn't support nurses if they're stressed or if something goes wrong."

Key Takeaways:

The rise of a culture that blames people for mistakes and the decline of a safe environment for people's mental well-being have severe implications for the NHS. This makes it hard for staff to perform their duties well, impacts the quality of care, and reduces the NHS's ability to improve continuously. This must be improved as a matter of urgency.

By understanding the issues, we can solve them.
Let there be hope!

3.4 Poor Teamwork, Alienation, and Loss of Professional Autonomy

The above problems naturally culminate in Poor Teamwork and loss of Professional Autonomy. These problems are deeply interrelated, feeding into and exacerbating each other, impacting the efficacy and morale of healthcare teams.

When staff members prioritise their survival[67] over working together, teamwork collapses. This creates a blame and fear culture, eroding trust and discouraging open communication. This breakdown in teamwork negatively affects the workplace atmosphere.

Professional autonomy is a critical issue in healthcare. To manage the complexities and risks involved in healthcare delivery, there is a tendency (especially with the problems identified above and reducing trust) to rely on standardisation and strict protocols. While guidelines are essential to ensure safety and quality, adhering too rigidly can stifle professional judgment and expertise. Worse, colleagues and patients can become dehumanised, which can even fan the flames of more significant division and even racism.[68]

---

67   i.e. this is beyond appropriate self-care due to dysfunctional systems
68   https://www.theguardian.com/society/2023/jul/10/racism-stain-nhs-royal-college-of-psychiatrists

What our network of nurses had to say on this issue:

"38 years I've been on that unit. Just because you're [now] on Bank and still doing the same job, you're not part of the team."

"You were expected to do more with less and for less, so you were just not getting the pay increase. You wouldn't get the support. And then if anything happened that was unsafe, or there was an incident, you wouldn't be ever backed up."

"It is difficult; they are being grumpy, ratty, and rude to their colleagues because they don't think their colleagues are working hard enough. And it's like, well, it's not for you to tell her whether she's working hard enough. You know, this sort of stuff."

"Then if it escalates and it's a big thing, you begin to manage someone, and then they come back with bullying. And it happens everywhere, you know. They come back saying they're not being treated fairly; it's very challenging."

"The other one is not tackling poor performance like lateness, sickness, etc. It's tackled by some people but not by others because they're perceived as too difficult. So again, that feeds into your team morale and how the team works. And then other people start thinking, well, it's my turn to get sick now because such and such has had her two weeks over Christmas."

"And by political, I mean, I'm really upset. That was because that doctor shouted at me in front of a patient in the ward. I'm upset because the nursing manager walked past me to go to the white nurse."

"I'm aware that internationally educated nurses get a bad deal. And it doesn't help when that isn't recognised or supported. For all sorts of complex reasons, like culture shock, racism, or not being given the support they need to flourish or being employed into jobs that are beneath their experience."

"But I think the other thing we see in the NHS is that it's too easy to go down the route of discipline. And discipline them for making a wrong decision, take them to task for what they did, or even dismiss them. But I supported them and said you made the right decision."

[Context of the nurse making the proper judgement, even though the outcome was unfortunate due to an extremely rare scenario.]

"There is racism throughout the NHS. Absolutely. People from ethnic minorities do not progress. They're not given the same opportunities. They are still a third more likely to be reported to the NMC[69] than their white colleagues. It is heart-wrenching, to be honest, because there are some fabulous people out there."

 Key Takeaways:

As you can see, things can quickly get ugly when things get tough. Poor teamwork, mistrust, and the loss of professional autonomy create a vicious cycle that further deteriorates the work environment and reduces job satisfaction. We must never forget that, ultimately, this all diminishes the quality of patient care.

By understanding the issues, we can solve them.
Let there be hope!

3.5   Poor Communication and Meetings

Exacerbated by the problems highlighted above and the lack of trust, the NHS typically struggles with communication and meetings. Meetings are often perceived merely as "moan-bonding events", which further lower morale rather than opportunities for constructive dialogue, problem-solving, and strategic planning. The resulting poor communication undermines the effectiveness of these meetings and contributes to a broader culture of inefficiency and dissatisfaction.

Meetings often waste time without clear objectives, actionable agendas, and effective facilitation. This can lead to participants feeling cynical about the organisation's ability to bring about change, which reduces the potential for meetings to serve as productive forums for identifying solutions, allocating resources, and aligning team efforts towards common goals.

---

69 Nursing and Midwifery Council (NMC)

Communication problems are common in the NHS. This reflects and reinforces the siloed operations of various departments or teams. When they fail to communicate effectively, important information is lost, misunderstandings occur, and it becomes difficult to coordinate patient care. This lack of communication leads to a lack of shared understanding and vision, weakening the organisation's collective response to challenges.

> 💬 **What our network of nurses had to say on this issue:**

"If you're working on the ward and you're short-staffed, it's very difficult to say I'm going to a clinical governance meeting because there's no one to look after the patients. So, there's something around sort of the unrealistic expectations of, like, what will you give up? I've given you the chance to come and talk at this meeting. But you've never been..." [Give up on meetings and governance because you can't leave patients, so communication suffers.]

"Nobody's listening, and it gets to the point: how many times can you keep saying it when no one's hearing it?"

"We are invited to participate in a consultation we can contribute to, but it's driven by us, not people seeking."

"The meetings I experience are moaning shops. Let's all get together and have a jolly good moan. It's usually about whoever is not in the room, which might be the management or healthcare assistants, and decide what we will take to the next meeting." [Not productive at all.]

"Going on maternity leave and coming back, and I've never had a year out before. And I came back, and oh my goodness. Can we go through everything? Tell me everything. She [my manager] went well, and the issues haven't changed. And she showed me this agenda, and I thought it was like complete déjà vu."

Ultimately, the issues of poor communication and unproductive meetings signify the levels of deep-rooted problems that the NHS face. Every meeting and form of communication must be an opportunity for fostering a culture of openness, collaboration, and continuous improvement. We will address how to do this in Section 4.

By understanding the issues, we can solve them.
Let there be hope!

3.6 Poor Understanding of Skill Mix and Optimal Role Structures

When healthcare teams lack a comprehensive understanding of the diverse skills and competencies required to provide quality patient care, it can lead to several issues. Tasks may be assigned inefficiently, staff capabilities may be underutilised, and workforce dynamics may be strained. This misalignment of skills can result in immediate and long-term consequences affecting patient care and organisational objectives.

Highly skilled professionals may do tasks that don't require their expertise, while less qualified people may be given complicated tasks they're unprepared for. This causes a waste of resources and prevents healthcare professionals from doing their best work. It can even lead to safety issues, job dissatisfaction and demotivation.

Clear role structures are essential for effective teamwork and collaboration. When roles and responsibilities are not well-defined, staff can experience confusion, inefficiencies, and conflicts. This can lead to overlap in duties or gaps in care, which can undermine the effectiveness of multidisciplinary teams and the safety of patients.

Although structures are essential because patient care is so complex, the greater the range of skills and capabilities, managed well, the more flexible the system can be to respond to specific patients and get the proper care delivered – first time.

What our network of nurses had to say on this issue:

"I think they are using them to replace nurses. So, whilst all the assistants are valuable, the trouble is they get used to them as a nurse replacement because they're cheaper to pay."

"You know, people are like, Oh, well, anyone can do that. We'll just give them a band 5."

"But there was no facility to do part-time work at that stage. It was somebody further up the food chain who said no. So, I couldn't match them on that at all. So, I thought I saw I've got no choice." [Retired early.]

"Well, nursing is the largest workforce and pay, but you can't do the job if it's not right. That goes for looking at everyone's role as well. As how many nurses you've got. You've got to understand the roles that go behind all those bands. I think they need to do some work on the front line to understand their areas and the challenges of those areas because there'll be differences from medical wards to surgical wards to A&E, care of the elderly, etc. They'll all have different challenges, and they'll all have different pinch points."

"You don't need a fixed career plan, but a goal of what you'd like to do and how you get there. And that's something that I think sometimes people struggle with. They think they can go from being a ward nurse for six months to a specialist nurse post without the expertise and experience required."

"We've also got lots of overseas nurses in the 54% of nurses registered with the NMC during that time last year. And that's a huge number of nurses we're bringing across. How nurses operate in other countries differs from average nurses and how their competence works in the UK. I think they're very reliant on permission to do things instead of having autonomy to do things."

Key Takeaways:

I would argue that people, especially nurses, are the NHS's greatest asset. However, the NHS is failing to optimise its skill mix and role structures, which is very costly to the nurses, NHS productivity, and quality of patient care. It can lead to delays in treatment, inconsistencies in care delivery, and an overall decline in patient satisfaction.

By understanding the issues, we can solve them.
Let there be hope!

3.7 Difficulty in Attracting and Retaining Staff and Professionalism

The NHS struggles to attract and keep employees due to many of the abovementioned issues. Among the issues are poor communication, an insufficient understanding of the skill mix, unmet demand for services, and a lack of professional autonomy. These problems create a challenging work environment that can deter potential employees and cause current staff to leave. The difficulty in finding and retaining new talent is a significant risk to the NHS's effectiveness and continuity.

Jobseekers hesitate to join organisations with a reputation for burnout, high workloads, and lack of support. The NHS, facing staff dissatisfaction and stress stories, struggles to compete for healthcare talent. The workforce may also seek better support, recognition, and professional growth opportunities elsewhere, including overseas.[70]

A lack of career development and advancement opportunities worsens the retention problem. A poor understanding of the best role structures and skill mixes causes this. When employees feel that their growth and contributions are limited or not valued, their commitment to the organisation decreases.

---

70 https://human-resources-health.biomedcentral.com/articles/10.1186/s12960-022-00789-y

The Financial Trap and Psychological Self-Protection

Those who can't find alternative employment that pays well enough to deal with their family commitments are "trapped". The financial constraints that many nurses face at home compel nurses to continue in their roles out of necessity rather than choice. This cohort (a significant one, typically in the middle of their career as the young can find other work and the experienced retire early) must resort to escaping through psychological protectionism.

The psychological impact of this financial trap is profound. Nurses describe how the intensity of their experiences, coupled with financial pressures, takes a toll on their mental health.

The only way for staff to deal with it and stay sane is to mentally "log out" and "go through the motions"; it's a form of absenteeism that must have profound implications.

💬 **What our network of nurses had to say on this issue:**

"I'm here because I have to be, not because I want to be."

"You're going through really traumatic experiences, you know, watching people die left, right and centre, and not being well cared for... your ability to cope with traumatic stuff is astonishing."

"When we're not at our best, the patients suffer."

"Nursing is one of the biggest jobs, with 27 million nurses worldwide. And now, we've got a recruiting crisis all over."

"The reason that nurses leave and feel burnt out is because they want to look after their patients well, and if it doesn't feel safe, and they don't feel they can..."

"There is so much negativity; the NHS is always in the news about the state of hospitals."

"I've got a friend who's a lecturer in nursing. When they were doing Zoom interviews, people would turn up to these Zoom interviews in their pyjamas and not take it as a professional interview."

"I just can't do this. Why do I do this? When I could go to Australia."

"The proactive, ambitious nurses who can make a real difference are usually quite good at what they do. They will not stay; they will seek something else."

"We're losing a hell of a lot of experience. Again, I have nothing against newly qualified nurses, but you can't expect someone through training to have the same experience when it's been about two years. We're losing experience, which we should use as role models for the younger nurses."

 Key Takeaways:

If we don't get the staffing right, the NHS will be a lost cause. It is important to note that these problems have far-reaching consequences beyond individual nurses. They affect patient care, team dynamics, and the entire healthcare system. This emphasises the need for a healthcare system that supports and nurtures its caregivers, as the well-being of nurses is directly linked to patient outcomes.

By understanding the issues, we can solve them. Let there be hope!

3.8   A Lack of Innovation and Improvement

When there is a high rate of workaround/rework, poor communication, excessive workloads, and difficulty in staff retention, it creates an environment where innovation and continuous improvement are not encouraged, as there is just too much firefighting. This lack of innovation is a big problem for the NHS because it prevents it from adapting to the changing needs of patients and advancements in managerial and medical technology.

The fear of being blamed for mistakes and the possibility of facing retribution discourages innovation and risk-taking. This leads to staff strictly following established protocols and procedures instead of proposing new solutions or ideas. This conservative approach is further amplified by high stress levels and burnout among healthcare professionals, leaving them with little motivation or energy to engage in creative problem-solving or advocate for improvements.

In addition, the NHS's siloed structure and poor communication channels prevent the effective sharing and implementation of new ideas across departments. This fragmentation makes it challenging to spread best practices and collaborate on innovations that could benefit the entire system.

The frequent staff turnover also makes it harder to develop new ideas. Experienced workers leave, and new employees struggle to adjust, disrupting the continuous improvement process. As we lose knowledge, progress becomes harder and harder to make.

 What our network of nurses had to say on this issue:

"That's the thing as well. We waste a lot of time in the NHS, reinventing the wheel for each. Each locality does its own thing when many of the ways we work are similar all around the country."

 Key Takeaways:

When there are so many dysfunctions, innovation falls to the bottom of nurses' agendas, while survival rises to the top. Out of all the interviews, there is very little conversation about innovation. The only reference I could find from over 150,000 words in the transcripts was this quote above.

By understanding the issues, we can solve them.
Let there be hope!

3.9   Poor Patient Care

As evidenced above, the NHS has many problems that affect patient care. As a result, patients often experience longer wait times, variations in the quality of care they receive, and an overall less satisfactory healthcare experience.

As evidenced earlier in the book, the demand for healthcare services is increasing, leading to longer wait times, less time for each patient, and lower quality of care. Communication issues can worsen these problems, leading to poor patient outcomes. Staff shortages also make it harder to provide high-quality care.

To make matters worse, the NHS is not keeping up with the latest advances in medical practice or healthcare delivery models[71], which means patients are missing out on the benefits. This is because the NHS is not innovating or continuously improving, causing a stagnation that reduces the efficiency and effectiveness of care. This also makes it difficult for the NHS to adapt to the changing needs and expectations of the people it serves.

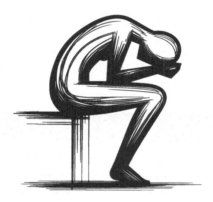

💬 **What our network of nurses had to say on this issue:**

"So our job is to get that many ops done that you discharged at that time, and if there's another problem, that will have to be dealt with by someone else! That's not nursing. That's not what the essence of nursing is about. And recently, I've been on the other side as a relative, and is it shocking how much of the basic care is missing?"

"I do believe it's because of targets. I mean, the nurses say they're really busy now, and I'm sure they are. I'm sure they're busy doing more because they're not busy doing basic care. Doing clerical

---

71 https://www.health.org.uk/publications/long-reads/international-comparisons-of-capital-in-health-care-why-is-the-uk-falling-behind

paperwork, you don't pick up scoring systems to check if people are deteriorating."

"My dad was in A&E. He was admitted with a clot in his lung. And we thought he got sepsis. So I've taken him in again, and they said, oh, no, he's not got a temperature. It's 36 something. So, the next day, I went in, and his temperature was 37.9. I said he's got an infection, and the response was – no, because he was not at 38 degrees. And I said, wait, it was only 36 yesterday. He's 92. He's been in bed all the time. No, because the rules say 38. He needed input immediately, but it didn't get acted upon." [The staff member was in a state of "computer says no" rather than using clinical judgement and critical thinking.]

"So, to the senior management boxes of 18 weeks – you can tick them which will satisfy that requirement but won't necessarily be in the patient's best interest."

"A disproportionate number of patients were dying from anti-cancer treatment because they were treated and then signposted to the GP or A&E – without the specialist expertise. And then, of course, they need to return to the place of specialists."

"For a tragic example of what we have been talking about, look up the Maddy Lawrence case[72] where a young girl was just ignored, seen as troublesome, and died."

 Key Takeaways:

The NHS faces significant challenges that undermine its core principle of providing comprehensive and accessible care to all. These issues have a cumulative effect that makes it difficult for the healthcare system to fulfil its mission, i.e. to serve patients. The NHS's reputation as a pillar of the UK's social welfare system is also at risk.

By understanding the issues, we can solve them.
Let there be hope!

---

72 https://www.bbc.co.uk/news/uk-england-bristol-66731277

Chapter 3 Summary

This chapter highlights the multiple challenges the NHS faces. The more we research, the more we can see how all these elements are interconnected.

The more the NHS can't cope, the more it "closes down" with dysfunctional targets and rules, and the more this happens, the less capable it becomes. Arguably, it is trapped in a cycle of decline, which fits very closely with the views of many interviewees who have been in the NHS for several decades but have never known it to be as challenging as this!

I believe there are ways to reverse this cycle. We will explain cognitive science in section three and the practical changes that can be made in section four. Before that, let's look at the symptoms of a troubled system. Are all these issues just academic hypotheses, or are they affecting the NHS in practice?

The challenges are tough, but there is hope and together the almost impossible is possible.

"Rather, ten times, die in the surf, heralding the way to a new world, than stand idly on the shore."
Florence Nightingale

Together for Tomorrow: Pioneering a New Era for the NHS

Signals and Evidence of a Failing System

Signals and Evidence of a Failing System Introduction

How can we tell if the problems highlighted in the previous three chapters are detrimental to nurses and the wider NHS, and if so, to what degree?

We need to look out for:

1. Widespread Burnout and Stress Among Staff
2. High Staff Turnover, Absenteeism and Dependency on temporary staff
3. Industrial Action
4. Staff Self-Neglect and "Emotional Log Out"
5. An Inability to Meet Targets Without Gaming the System
6. Over-reliance on Reports, Inspections and Audits
7. Patient Dissatisfaction, Complaints and Poorer Outcomes

4.1 Widespread Burnout and Stress Among Staff

Recent studies and surveys paint a troubling picture of the mental health and well-being of healthcare professionals across the NHS.

A 2020 British Medical Association (BMA) survey found that 58% of doctors reported higher stress levels than before the pandemic, with burnout rates alarmingly on the rise.[73] The BMJ reported in 2021 that nearly half of NHS staff in England have reported feeling unwell from work-related stress, and a significant portion are considering quitting their jobs.[74] These findings underscore the immense pressure and mental strain that NHS staff are under, exacerbated by the challenges discussed earlier, including overwhelming workloads, inadequate support, and a culture often prioritising bureaucratic compliance over staff welfare.

The NHS Staff Survey of 2020 revealed that nearly 44% of staff reported feeling unwell due to work-related stress in the last 12 months, the highest figure recorded in five years.[75]

---

73 https://www.bma.org.uk/media/5620/20220141-bma-COVID-19 Pandemic-review-report-2-the-impact-of-the-pandemic-on-the-medical-profession-final.pdf#:~:text=URL%3A%20 https%3A%2F%2Fwww.bma.org.uk%2Fmedia%2F5620%2F20220141

74 https://www.bmj.com/content/372/bmj.n703

75 https://www.bmj.com/content/372/bmj.n703

And in the staff survey of 2022[76] the key statistics are:

Work-Related Stress: 44.8% of staff reported feeling unwell due to work-related stress in the last 12 months, indicating significant stress among NHS employees.

Burnout and Emotional Exhaustion:

46.3%	of staff feel worn out at the end of their working day/shift.
39.9%	report that their work frustrates them.
37.4%	find their work emotionally exhausting.
34.0%	feel burnt out because of their work.

Harassment, Bullying, and Abuse

27.8%	of staff experienced at least one incident of harassment, bullying, or abuse from patients, service users, their relatives, or other public members.
11.1%	experienced it from managers.
18.7%	experienced it from other colleagues.

These statistics are not just numbers; they are a call for help from NHS staff. The evidence is clear: the systemic problems troubling the NHS are diminishing its operational efficiency and jeopardising the health and well-being of its most valuable asset – its workforce.

💬 **What our network of nurses had to say on this issue:**

"I remember that year, and I would go to bed at night after a long shift. I actively remember closing my eyes and hearing the alarms going off and hearing the monitors, and I would get into that and count at night. Okay, I'm only going to have six hours of sleep. I'm going to have five

---

76 https://www.nhsstaffsurveys.com/results/national-results/

hours, but it's okay. I can get through 13 hours tomorrow, and it will be okay. So, it was a sense of just kind of survival mode."

"So when the doctors feel as though they're being pulled left, right and centre and there are not enough of them to get to everything that they needed to, which is awful, but it's the nurses, the ones on the ward with those ten patients who are deteriorating that are struggling. You can't do anything, and you have nowhere to go, and you're watching these people deteriorating before your eyes, and you can't do anything about it; the burden is a different but very heavy one."

"I've been a nurse for 24 or 25 years. And she went on [therapist], it's taken you this long to have a breakdown. And I remember thinking, oh my god, you know, and I look around like my life; my dad was a nurse, and he had had a breakdown. It's almost the accepted thing that nurses go through."

"When people get very burnt out, they're being prevented from doing what's in line with their values."

 Key Takeaways:

This last quote is very powerful and insightful. When operating in line with your meaning you can manage almost anything. Viktor Frankl is a great inspiration (his logotherapy is all about finding meaning), and he was a guiding light to us all as he managed to survive and stay positive through five Nazi concentration camps! You can often make the impossible possible when you have meaning! However, this is not to say that we don't need to tackle burnout and stress; we do.

By understanding the issues, we can solve them.
Let there be hope!

4.2 High Staff Turnover, Absenteeism and Dependency on Temporary Staff

The NHS faces a critical workforce shortage, with an alarming 124,000 full-time equivalent (FTE) staff vacancies reported in NHS trusts as of December 2022. The situation is particularly dire for nursing positions, which account for over a third of all vacancies. This highlights the urgent need to address the acute shortfall. The staff leaver rate in NHS trusts has also risen from 9.6% in the year to September 2020, to 12.5% in September 2022, with the leaver rate for NHS nurses and health visitors increasing from 9% to 11.5% during the same period. This trend is concerning, especially as the NHS aims to reduce the nursing vacancy rate to 5% by 2028, according to The Health Foundation.

Moreover, a record number of NHS staff, particularly nurses, have expressed feeling "truly broken"[77]. In quarter two of last year, 42,400 staff voluntarily quit their NHS jobs, marking the highest departure rate over a decade. The primary reasons cited for resigning include seeking better pay and work-life balance, with a significant number of staff leaving for "a better reward package", highlighting the urgent need for the NHS to address these issues to retain its workforce (The Independent).

Detailed workforce statistics can be found here.[78]

💬 **What our network of nurses had to say on this issue:**

"For workers, there's just no way forward. They see it as a bottomless pit and can't see a solution. Therefore, they can't even grip and control their self-care, and I feel awful. Every day. I can't get out of the cycle. Just in that space at the moment, like I can't do this. I'm running out of resilience sharpish and must find a job elsewhere. I've been going to bed earlier at night and then just suffering with a helicopter mind. Fighting and wanting to make it work. That's the cycle."

"Lots of friends have become very bitter. Very disengaged, have left because they've just had enough."

"Because you haven't got access to what you need to provide this best standard of care, which is what you're taught at university. So, you come in, and you've got this sense that I'm not doing what I should be. I'm not doing the best I can; I've been told that I'm supposed to provide this best practice of care, and I can't. So, I think that also has a psychological impact."

77 https://www.independent.co.uk/news/health/nhs-staff-resign-record-b2261689.html
78 https://digital.nhs.uk/data-and-information/publications/statistical/nhs-workforce-statistics/october-2023

"That's a real worry. The retention of nurses. Yeah, we're losing so much experience all the time."

"My kids sat me down. They were like, Mum, where are you going? Now? You've got to get out of what you're doing, the number of hours you're working, and holding everything together, but then you feel if you go, who will they replace you with?"

 Key Takeaways:

Every NHS leader must prioritise staff retention as there is evidently a material problem. Although pay is undoubtedly an issue, all the variables within section one of this book need careful consideration and proactive management, including teamwork and finding meaning and purpose, i.e. becoming a "Patient Champion".

By understanding the issues, we can solve them.
Let there be hope!

4.3   Industrial Action

The NHS has experienced significant industrial action in recent years, marking an unprecedented phase of disputes over pay, working conditions, and the impact of staffing shortages exacerbated by soaring inflation and pandemic backlogs. In December 2022, more than 10,000 ambulance workers across nine NHS trusts in England and Wales voted to strike, leading to two 24-hour strikes. Similarly, UNISON members and more than 1,600 Unite the Union workers in various ambulance services participated in strikes, pointing to widespread discontent among NHS staff.[79] These actions underscore the critical tensions between healthcare workers and government pay offers. The most significant strike within the NHS occurred on 6 February 2023, coinciding with nurse strikes (Wikipedia).

The junior doctors' strikes, particularly notable for their scale and impact, further illustrate the depth of the crisis. The British Medical Association (BMA) highlighted a demand for pay restoration to 2008 levels, citing real-

---

79   https://www.unison.org.uk/news/press-release/2022/12/unison-ambulance-workers-strike-over-pay-and-staffing/

term pay cuts of nearly 30% since then. A significant ballot in February 2023 saw more than 98% of junior doctors voting for strike action, leading to a 72-hour strike in March that disrupted an estimated 175,000 appointments and procedures. Despite attempts at negotiation, further strikes were announced, including a historic 96-hour strike, emphasising the deadlock between healthcare workers and the government.[80]

In England, the NHS braced for "the most disruptive industrial action" in its history as junior doctors walked out over pay and working conditions. The four-day walkout was predicted to postpone up to a quarter of a million appointments, with the NHS Confederation warning of a "catastrophic impact" on the NHS's capacity (The Journal[81]).

"Across the NHS, we have now seen more than half a million appointments and procedures rescheduled over the last six months as a result of strikes from staff in a range of NHS roles – and with each strike, it is becoming harder. Our staff are doing all they possibly can to manage the disruption and deliver rescheduled appointments as quickly as possible, but there's no doubt that each round of industrial action makes it more difficult for the NHS to tackle the backlog." Deputy chief nurse Charlotte McArdle.

At the time of writing, we have seen industrial action across the NHS that has impacted more than a million hospital appointments.

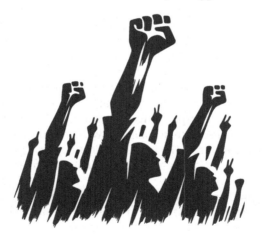

---

80   https://www.bmj.com/content/380/bmj.p701

81   https://www.thejournal.ie/england-nhs-industrial-action-junior-doctors-6041155-Apr2023/

What our network of nurses had to say on this issue:

"At the end of the day, some harm comes to the patient under your care, and it's you in court. It's not the directors; it's your registration when something goes wrong, and I don't think nurses want that on their conscience."

"We haven't got enough people. No one's listening. So, either I can get on with it, or I'm just stepping away because I disagree with it. And I think that's where nurses are now; they have gotten to the point where they don't want to be complicit in the poor management and what happens to patients. Unless they strike against it, they look as guilty as the people allowing it."

"Nurses are bringing trauma and stress from home into work due to chronic underfunding and low pay. This impacts their ability to provide compassionate care. Nurses have been chronically underfunded and underpaid for years."

 Key Takeaways:

My view is that industrial action is not driven primarily by pay. As seen in this section of the book, many are exhausted and frustrated with the system, and the main concern is patient safety. It seems apparent that the system is not operating optimally, and we must take action to fix it.

By understanding the issues, we can solve them. Let there be hope!

4.4   Self-Neglect and Emotionally Logged Out

Self-Neglect: The Sacrifice in Caring

Nursing requires a lot of effort and selflessness, which can sometimes lead to nurses neglecting their own needs. It's important to remember that taking care of yourself is just as crucial as taking care of others. Not looking after your own basic needs can cause physical exhaustion and mental and emotional health issues. This can lead to a cycle of self-neglect that can ultimately affect the quality of care that patients receive.

The consequences of this are significant and can have many different effects. Extended periods of self-neglect can lead to burnout. It can sneak up on a nurse and make it harder for them to feel compassion and empathy, which is why they come to work in the first place. Burnout can cause a nurse to feel disconnected from the job they once loved and turn them into a disillusioned employee just going through the motions.

Emotionally Logged Out: The Invisible Shield

Nurses often dissociate emotionally as a coping mechanism to help them deal with the constant stress of the job. This detachment is a cause for concern as it indicates a deeper issue – a lack of passion and commitment to their work as a survival mechanism.

This trend reflects the widespread disillusionment within the nursing profession. Emotional withdrawal can lead to bitterness and disengagement and even cause many nurses to leave the profession prematurely. This is worrying and is already leading to a catastrophic loss of experienced nurses.

This trend also affects inexperienced nurses. They often struggle to cope with the reality of working in a ward, where they find that the practices they learned through qualification do not align with the actual work. This leads to a lack of confidence and questions about their career choice.

A young nurse shared her experience of loving her training, but soon after starting work on the ward, she began looking for a way out. She experienced pre-shift anxiety, which made her dread going to work. Fortunately, she found a job in specialist nursing, where the system was better, management was better, and patient care was great – exactly what she wanted to be part of. She loved nursing again. It is important to note that the core problem is often not with the nurses' empathy and compassion, but with the system letting nurses down.

The interviews revealed that nursing can be both great and terrible. It's wonderful when nurses can provide excellent care to patients. However, when factors outside their control, like system failures, prevent them from helping needy patients, it can be incredibly stressful and frustrating. Some nurses feel they must leave their jobs as a result. Many nurses are leaving the NHS to work in healthcare in Australia, or to find alternative employment.

Mental health support for healthcare workers is also lacking. Many professionals feel that their own emotional and psychological needs are often overlooked. This leads to a workforce frequently under immense stress, with limited avenues for relief.

What our network of nurses had to say on this issue:

"I don't even have time to think about myself."

"I can see with my young colleague that she doesn't have that emotional barrier yet. So, she works extra hours and is very submissive to consultants. She wants to please everybody, which again, you know, we tried to tell her gently about having boundaries, and I think she's just starting to realise that it's not sustainable to work at that level."

"Skipping meals has become a norm; there's just no time."

"Managing poor behaviour or poor performance, which inevitably results from not feeling valued and not feeling like you're able to do your job properly. So, you know, feeling resentful about it, and then it causes problems."

"I just go through the motions now."

"I see that happening all the time. People coming in do their job as little as they can because that's how they can help preserve their personal inside. Just doing the minimum, yeah. I'm not there. I do think when you're emotionally locked out, then you can't provide the care you want to provide. So that, again, in itself is a bit of a vicious cycle."

"They just don't have that fuel; they want to carry on and do things. Another escape, I think linked to depression, is poor eating or drinking because it's a release for them."

4.5   Inability to Meet Targets Without Gaming the System

Three of the most high-profile targets are waiting times for elective treatment, waiting times for being seen in A&E and waiting times for cancer services.

Over the past number of years, the data shows that, in general, performance has been declining across the board.

High waits for treatment are not new. Before the pandemic in February 2020 there were already 4.43 million people on a waiting list for care.

The figures for December 2023 show:[82]

- The waiting list is 7.60 million cases, consisting of approximately 6.37 million individual patients waiting for treatment.
- Around 3.30 million of these patients have been waiting more than 18 weeks;
- Over 337,000 patients have been waiting more than a year for treatment.

---

82 https://www.bma.org.uk/advice-and-support/nhs-delivery-and-workforce/pressures/nhs-backlog-data-analysis

- A median waiting time for treatment of 15 weeks – almost double the pre-COVID-19 Pandemic median wait of 8.3 weeks in December 2019.

The NHS Constitution sets out principles and values for the NHS, patients' rights, and what they can expect from the NHS. This includes the right for patients to access certain services within maximum waiting times.

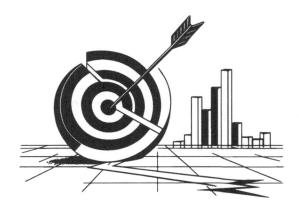

Elective treatment[83]

Elective or planned treatment generally refers to procedures scheduled in advance, e.g. a hip replacement, removing a mole or cataract surgery.

Since 2009, the target for elective treatment has been that at least 92% of patients begin treatment within 18 weeks of being referred from a GP to a specialist. The NHS has not met this target since February 2016.

More people are receiving elective treatment. Higher demand for treatment means the number of people on the waiting list is also growing. The waiting list for elective treatment in April 2012 was 2.5 million; by March 2019, this had risen to around 4.2 million.

Elective treatment is affected by changes in medical practice and increased demand. Medical advances mean more people can be treated; for example, the number of day surgery cases has risen in recent years, reducing the need for overnight stays and allowing more patients to be treated.

83   https://www.futurelearn.com/info/courses/the-nhs-explained/0/
steps/47867#:~:text=The%20NHS%20has%20a%20number,like%20x%2Drays%20or%20scans.

Accident and emergency (A&E)[84]

The target for A&E waiting times states that at least 95% of patients should be seen within four hours. In the NHS in England, A&E services have not met this target since July 2015.

Rising demand is part of the challenge of meeting the A&E waiting times target, and we also know that increasing numbers of patients attending A&E have multiple health conditions and are more likely to be admitted to hospital.

In addition to increasing demand, waiting times in A&E have been affected by a squeeze on hospital resources. The number of hospital beds has decreased by 4% since 2011/12, and the percentage of occupied beds has risen from 89% to 92%.

Cancer[85]

There are several targets for accessing cancer treatment. The NHS's priority for cancer is that at least 85% of patients diagnosed with cancer should begin treatment within 62 days of an urgent referral from their GP.

This target was introduced in 2009 and was met for several years; however, this target has not been met at a national level since 2013/14. Despite this, there has been a rise in the number of patients beginning cancer treatment within two months, from around 116,000 in 2012/13 to approximately 150,000 in 2018/19.

 What our network of nurses had to say on this issue:

"Our targets have gone through the roof because we weren't operating for two or three years [COVID-19 Pandemic]. So now, for example, our waiting list was one year; it's now two years. So, there's a push for the managers to get that back down because the government says you need to operate on people within this time.

---

84 https://www.futurelearn.com/info/courses/the-nhs-explained/0/
steps/47867#:~:text=The%20NHS%20has%20a%20number,like%20x%2Drays%20or%20scans.

85 https://www.futurelearn.com/info/courses/the-nhs-explained/0/
steps/47867#:~:text=The%20NHS%20has%20a%20number,like%20x%2Drays%20or%20scans.

There's no extra resource, and professionals involved in that care are on their knees as they're already doing extra care."

"There is a loss of focus on the patient. Organisations focus on operational targets rather than quality and safety."

"Managers often don't listen to frontline nursing staff and prioritise targets over patient care."

For more details on the potential dysfunctions of targets, please see Appendix 2.

 Key Takeaways:

The NHS is not meeting its targets. It's well known that human beings game systems and report to meet targets, but the NHS is still not meeting targets, and it's getting increasingly worse every year. An argument could be made that things are so challenging that focusing on narrow targets no longer works, and there is nowhere to hide.

Focusing on waiting list targets through practices that help numerical goals are often at the expense of patient service quality. This can include prioritising treatments based on target metrics over medical urgency, or using administrative strategies to meet waiting time targets without enhancing patient care. This might make it look better on paper, but it worsens the care of patients.

By understanding the issues, we can solve them. Let there be hope!

4.6   Patient Dissatisfaction, Complaints and Poorer Outcomes

The King's Fund summarises this very well with their reporting on the "Public satisfaction with the NHS and social care in 2022".[86]

---

86 https://www.kingsfund.org.uk/insight-and-analysis/reports/public-satisfaction-nhs-and-social-care-2022

Results from the British Social Attitudes survey:

Customer satisfaction with the NHS in 2022 has declined significantly. The overall satisfaction rate has dropped by seven percentage points from 2021 to 29%. This is the lowest level of satisfaction recorded since the survey started in 1983. More than half of the respondents (51%) expressed dissatisfaction with the NHS, the highest percentage recorded since the survey began.

The decrease in satisfaction was uniform across all age groups, income levels, genders, and supporters of different political parties. The primary reason for dissatisfaction with the NHS was waiting times for GP and hospital appointments (69%), followed by staff shortages (55%) and the belief that the government does not spend enough money on the NHS (50%).

Of those who were satisfied with the NHS, the primary reason was that NHS care is free at the point of use (74%), followed by the quality of NHS care (55%), and the availability of a wide range of services and treatments (49%).

 What our network of nurses had to say on this issue:

"What will the impact be on people? When my dad got discharged, and I said, what about this incontinence thing, now that you think he's now incontinent? Oh, well, he's ready for discharge, and you'll have to talk to the GP about that. It's like not my problem. But it should be your problem because he will end up back in your hospital."

Key Takeaways:

After reviewing all the transcripts and coding, I was surprised to find limited explicit quotes regarding complaints and poor patient experience. However, from all the interviews, it is clear that nurses' #1 priority is patient care. The hypothesis is that nurses are implicitly pointing out patient experiences. I also expect that there will be a considerable amount of "emotional log out", as discussed earlier. Nonetheless, the national surveys and statistics indicate an evident deterioration, another transparent signal that the NHS system is seriously troubled.

By understanding the issues, we can solve them.
Let there be hope!

Chapter 4 Summary

Throughout this chapter, we have examined various indicators of a dysfunctional system in the healthcare industry. These include burnout, difficulties in recruitment and retention, industrial action, self-neglect and emotional exhaustion, an inability to hit targets, and patient dissatisfaction. While each of these signals is significant, it becomes clear that the NHS system requires fundamental reform when viewed holistically. Making only minor adjustments will not be sufficient to fix it.

"For perhaps the first time since the industrial revolution, health factors are acting as a serious headwind to UK economic growth. They are contributing significantly to a shrinking labour force and stalling productivity."[87] Andy Haldane, former Chief Economist at the Bank of England.

Nurses, Midwives, and Allied Health Professionals need to be the foundation of the revolution, and we will explore this in section four of the book.

---

87 https://99-percent.org/the-rational-policy-makers-guide-to-the-nhs-at-holyrood/

Mental Shortcut.

We will cover Mental Shortcuts in section 3; in the meantime, please take from section 1 that the NHS is very difficult to manage, and we should not blame or demonise any group within the NHS (especially managers); we need to be in this together; we need to propel the 2nd Positive Healthcare Revolution together.

The challenges are tough, but there is hope and together the almost impossible is possible.

"I think one's feelings waste themselves in words; they ought all to be distilled into actions which bring results."
Florence Nightingale

Together for Tomorrow: Pioneering a New Era for the NHS

The Vision for Where We Want to Get To

Part 1 provides a challenging view of the NHS's current situation. This understanding is crucial because we can't determine where we stand without it and chart a course for progress.

Similarly, when we're caught up in solving problems each day, it's easy to lose sight of our ultimate goals and what success looks like. This section is essential because it allows us to reach a consensus on what we aim to achieve and set expectations that we can all strive towards.

Chapter 5

Our End Goals / Vision

5.1   The Vision for Nurses:

In an ideal yet realistic healthcare scenario, our nurse's day begins with a smooth, well-organised start to their shift. They are empowered and supported, buoyed by a system that values their expertise and dedication to patient care. Their organisation embraces a culture of innovation, where nurses are encouraged and equipped to seek out and implement new ways to enhance patient outcomes, i.e. to be **"Patient Champions".** This forward-thinking environment is matched by a management team that sees nurses as the **foundation of change** and sees its primary role as enabling nurses to excel, offering support, resources, and encouragement to pursue innovative solutions.

Our nurse experiences a harmonious blend of technology and personal touch throughout the day, where innovative tools enhance patient care without replacing the human element. They engage in their duties with confidence and purpose, bolstered by technology that simplifies administrative tasks and enriches patient interactions. Patients are active participants in their care, equipped with educational and empowering tools. The environment is calm and healing, designed with input from the whole team of healthcare professionals to ensure functionality and comfort.

In our ideal NHS, nurses go beyond the routine tasks of managing patients and channel their rich experience and intuition to deliver exceptional care. They embody the spirit of proactive healthcare, using their insights to anticipate patient needs and prevent complications before they arise. This intuitive approach allows for a more personalised and responsive care model, where the nurse's judgement plays a critical role in reducing unnecessary medical interventions. In this light, nursing is not just about responding to health crises.

At the end of the shift our nurses discuss 'What went well', 'What didn't go well' and 'What can we learn for tomorrow'.

Nurses are fundamental in shaping a healthcare system that emphasises preventative care, enhancing patient outcomes and overall system efficiency. This additional layer of expertise and foresight positions nursing at **the core of a proactive, patient-centred healthcare system**; at the core of the **Second Positive Healthcare Revolution.**

The nurse takes breaks in a well-appointed staff lounge that promotes relaxation and camaraderie. Professional development opportunities are woven into their routine, with access to in-house training and external mentorship programmes that encourage career growth and innovation. Leadership is visible and supportive, fostering a culture of continuous improvement and well-being.

Nurses focus on patients' well-being and provide nurturing care that promotes safety, comfort, and trust. This approach creates a healing environment that empowers patients and equips them with the knowledge they need to take control of their health. Our nurse's commitment to treating every patient with dignity and compassion at every step ensures patients leave feeling supported and inspired to take responsibility for their health.

As the day concludes, our nurses reflect on the positive impacts they have made and the lives they have impacted, feeling a profound sense of satisfaction and pride in their work. They leave work with a smile and a spring in their step. In this ideal healthcare system, nursing is not just a job; it's a calling, celebrated and supported in every aspect. In such an environment, nursing becomes the best job in the world, embodying a perfect blend of compassion, innovation, and excellence.

5.2   The Vision for Patients:

Imagine a patient named Emma who is going through the healthcare system. She starts by visiting her GP for a health issue concerning her. As soon as she enters the primary care facility (within days, not weeks), she feels a sense of warmth and attention, which immediately eases her anxiety. Her GP listens to her attentively and uses their medical expertise and compassion to set the tone for a healthcare experience that values her as an individual, not just a case number.

As Emma moves on to secondary care[88] for further treatment, she notices that her GP and hospital specialists communicate seamlessly, ensuring that her care is personal and comprehensive. Every professional is current on her case, and the hospital environment is characterised by efficiency and empathy, further alleviating her fears. Nurses and doctors take the time to explain procedures, answer questions, and offer reassurance, making Emma feel genuinely seen and supported. Emma receives responsive care tailored to her needs throughout her

---

88 Could equally be a direct to community care scenario – equally as efficient

hospital stay, focusing on her comfort and well-being. The nursing staff's caring gestures and advanced treatment technologies foster a healing atmosphere that significantly contributes to her recovery.

When Emma returns to the community for long-term management, she finds a support network waiting for her. Care teams and community health workers continue the compassionate care she received in the hospital, focusing on her recovery and quality of life. This ongoing support helps her feel confident and secure in managing her health, with accessible resources and guidance every step of the way. Reflecting on her journey, Emma feels deeply grateful for the healthcare system and the professionals who guided her. She marvels at the difference responsive, patient-centred care made in her recovery and outlook on health.

The system, designed to heal and support, has given her better health outcomes and a renewed trust and appreciation for healthcare. Emma noticed a remarkable difference in her healthcare experience, with no prolonged waits or delays, thanks to a highly efficient system powered by innovations that nurses have spearheaded with a patient-centric approach.

Every transition from primary to secondary care and back into community management was smooth, with no gaps in her treatment or care coordination. This efficiency is vital for Emma, who manages a long-term condition requiring consistent monitoring and care. The system's agility and responsiveness mean that her condition is managed proactively, with regular check-ins and adjustments to her care plan as needed, all without the stress of waiting or feeling lost in the system.

Emma's journey reflects a healthcare system that prioritises patient needs and outcomes, where efficiency and compassion go hand in hand. This significantly enhances her quality of life and gives her confidence in managing her health. The emphasis on swift, effective care, driven by the innovative spirit of nursing professionals, showcases a healthcare model driven by nurses as "Patient Champions" that truly puts patients first.

5.3   The Vision for NHS Managers:

Meet James, an NHS manager passionate about creating a work environment that fosters innovation and teamwork. Unlike many managers who focus solely on meeting top-down targets, James believes empowering nurses and frontline staff is the key to improving patient care and increasing system efficiency (with the side effect of improving his targets). He recognises the invaluable insights and experiences that nurses and frontline staff bring and greatly emphasises their contributions to healthcare delivery.

James has witnessed the impact of giving nurses a voice[89] and allowing them to share ideas and solutions. He has seen how this empowers them and leads to tangible improvements in patient care and operational workflows. James is committed to facilitating forums and systems where staff can express their concerns and suggest innovative ideas to transform the healthcare delivery system.

By adopting this approach, James has transformed the culture within his department, creating a place where every team member feels valued and heard. He has shifted his focus from chasing retrospective targets to leading a forward-thinking department where collaboration and continuous improvement drive excellence. This shift has made James's role more fulfilling and rewarding, while contributing to better patient outcomes and a more resilient and sustainable NHS.

5.4   Summary – The Gap That We Must Bridge

Thanks to the stark analysis in section 1 and the vision in section 2, we now have a clear view of the gap we must close. There is a strong tension between sections one and two, and that has been the planned intention of this book. Only through this tension can you "feel" the strength of will to facilitate such change.

Most people will see this tension in one of two ways:

1.   Great, let's do this; let's work together and make a dent[90] in the NHS
2.   This is impossible, it just can't be done

My belief is that such transformations can be made without the need for radically increased budgets. There will be a need for seed funding to support the changes, but fundamentally, finance should not be seen as

---

89 He often utilises www.Insigt-Genie.com for this knowledge capture.

90 With reference to the famous Steve Jobs quote about Apple making big changes

the barrier to change, i.e. it should not be part of the "this can't be done" excuse mindset.

To those whose mental frame is in the second camp, I urge you to practise an open mind and to study the following sections carefully. I hope the book will make a "dent"[91] in your cognition; humans working together can achieve great things.

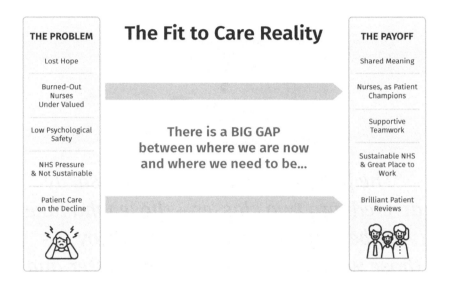

However, before we rush to the solutions in Section Four, Section Three explores the cognitive and behavioural science behind WHY we consistently fall into the problems identified in Section One. The next section is crucial for our understanding and lays the foundation and new language for successful change. Don't miss Section Three!

---

91 With reference to the famous Steve Jobs quote about Apple making big changes

"The progressive world is necessarily divided into two classes – those who take the best of what there is and enjoy it – those who wish for something better and try to create it." **Florence Nightingale**

Together for Tomorrow: Pioneering a New Era for the NHS

The Science and Insights That Explain the Problems

Science and Insights Introduction – The Importance of Cognitive and Behavioural Science

Overwhelm is a human condition that affects us all, particularly today with modern technology and social media. Even though our brains are amazing, and we have the highest cognitive ability of all life on earth, we still get overwhelmed by the amount of information thrown at us – especially in the NHS!

Section 3 will summarise the cognitive challenges we face, how our brains cope, and the problems we face. We will use these concepts for the practical solutions in Section 4.

The good news is that when we understand these constraints and how our brains work, there are simple things that we can do to reduce stress, reduce errors, and improve all our lives.

These concepts are the root cause of most problems/constraints/misunderstandings in your life – both with loved ones at home and colleagues at work.

Over the last three years, I have spent much of my life studying and applying these insights. They have changed my life, and my vision is for them to significantly improve your life, too.

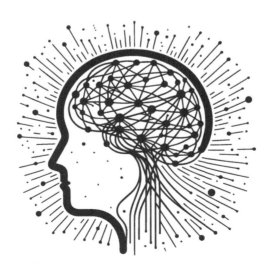

Chapter 6

Overwhelm

6.1 Overwhelm – the general understanding.

I would be very surprised if **all** nurses reading this book didn't feel a connection to the word "overwhelm" when working in the NHS. This word is also very strongly featured in Section 1.

We all know this general feeling of being overwhelmed by too much to do and insufficient hours in the day. The aftereffects can be devastating; in the introduction, sickness rates, vacancies, and mental health deterioration are all linked. Many dysfunctions within the NHS drive much of this general overwhelm.

However, let's explore how your brain manages overwhelm from a cognitive science perspective. Without this level of understanding, we are unable to generate solutions to the problems and dysfunctions of the NHS, i.e. this knowledge is critical.

The following pages should spark several lightbulb moments for you. We need you to commit these insights to memory, as you will see how they apply to many problems (day in and day out) in your personal and professional life.

6.2 Mental Overwhelm – how your brain works.

The first insight I want to share is called combinatory explosion (previously touched upon in chapter two in The Perils of Over-Siloed, Over-Simplified Systems section), or we can call it **Mental Overwhelm,** from now on to simplify the language. And the best way to illustrate this concept is with a chess example, as mentioned in chapter two.

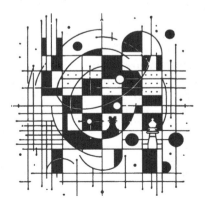

You can see on the chess board that there are 32 pieces, and on average, there are 30 possible legal moves per play in a game of chess, and on average, 60 moves per game. Therefore, if you do the maths on this, i.e. 30 to the power 60, this generates such a vast number that there are more potential outcomes, just on a game of chess, than there are particles in the Universe,[92] which is incredible. It's so incredible it's hard to comprehend. The number is so vast that even the most powerful computers can't possibly compute it, certainly not in a timeframe that you could play a game of chess!

 Reflect

Take a moment to make sense of this insight and what it means. Today, considering colleagues, patients, people you encounter travelling and family members, you might well deal with more than 32 people (equate to the chess pieces). Each of these has many more rules than the chess pieces, i.e. drivers (values, religion, preferences, etc.) and constraints (time, resources, medical conditions, etc.) So, I argue that there are more possible outcomes and decisions that you are bombarded with – every day – than there are particles in the universe.

 Insight

This is why strict rules and checklists CAN NEVER serve a health department in isolation – they should only ever be guidelines. Ultimately, healthcare professionals must be well-trained and have the autonomy to overrule simplistic checklists where appropriate. Remember back in Section 1, the examples of checklist management gone wrong ("Computer Says No" type management) where infection was not managed due to the temperature being 0.1 degrees off protocol (despite all the other relevant variables). Plus, pain relief was not given to a 92-year-old man with several broken ribs because it had not been four hours since his last paracetamol, even though he had not had the maximum possible dose. Simple rules and checklists can never adequately direct treatment and care in such a complex environment; they can only be support guides. There are too many variables for checklists to cover.

---

92 Professor John Vervaeke – YouTube series Awakening from the Meaning Crisis https://www.youtube.com/playlist?list=PLND1JCRq8Vuh3f0P5qjrSdb5eC1ZfZwWJ

If the scale of complexity within your job does not blow your mind, then it would be worth a re-read of this section.

So, how does our brain cope with this level of information and manage against mental overwhelm?

Overall, it does an outstanding job.

The answer is "heuristics", which could be called the Rules of Thumb. From now on, we will refer to this concept as a **Mental Shortcut.**

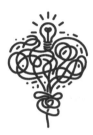

Our brains are very good at identifying patterns in this mass of information. For example, a patient could theoretically ask for a drink from hundreds of options (different drinks: milk/no milk, sugar/no sugar, extra water to cool, etc.). Imagine having to check every possible requirement for every patient every time... Instead, the patient (and you learn) uses mental shortcuts to say, "Tea, two sugars and milk, please", and you will typically get to know that the choice usually boils down to a few rather than hundreds (thankfully).

With more than 35,000 daily decisions,[93] we must use these mental shortcuts to get through life. Otherwise, we become overwhelmed. And you'd go insane if you had to deal with the quantity and volume of information that hits us every day.

A lot of language developed over the last two and a half thousand years gives us the impression that there's an absolute science and absolute algorithm to give us absolute answers. But as you can see, with the chess example, that is not possible; it's not true that there is an absolute answer/algorithm for many things – certainly not one that is practical. We MUST use mental shortcuts.

---

93 Roberts Wesleyan College's resource on strategic leadership https://go.roberts.edu/ leadingedge/the-great-choices-of-strategic-leaders

How We Manage The World Around Us

Information Overwhelm

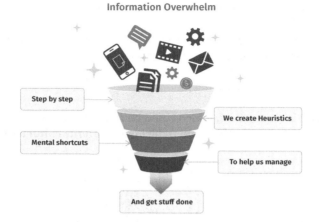

6.3 "Mental Shortcuts" Seem Great – What's The Problem?

Henry Priest's book Biased – 50 Powerful Cognitive Biases illustrates many of the most common biases. I believe that most of these 50 biases are linked to the concept of Mental Overload. When we use Mental Shortcuts in the wrong place, context, or time, they are no longer Mental Shortcuts that help us – they are Biases that could (and often do) lead to significant error/harm.

Not only do we use mental shortcuts frequently (almost half of what we do is habitual[94]), but we are not even conscious that we are using them.

For example, you have been dealing with a ward of ten patients for a month, and over the last few days, one patient, Gladys, has required more pain relief than usual.

If a ward manager asked you, "Over the last month, which patient has been in the most discomfort?" you might well answer Gladys because your recent exposure/data recall comes to mind first (Availability Bias). The amount of accurate, detailed data for all patients over a month is too much to comprehend, and we often fall foul of Mental Shortcuts, giving us the wrong answers.

---

94 "Habits in Everyday Life: Thought, Emotion, and Action" by Wendy Wood, Jeffrey M. Quinn, and Deborah A. Kashy, published in 2002. This study suggested that about 43% of daily behaviours are performed out of habit.

I'm sure you can now see how we can fall into dangerous traps with Mental Shortcuts if we are not careful.

 Takeaways To Remember:

1. The volume of data hitting your brain is mentally overwhelming – Every day
2. We MUST use Mental Shortcuts all the time
3. We must always be mindful through reflection that we are not falling into the Bias Traps that we can fall into with these Mental Shortcuts.

Mental Overwhelm

Summary

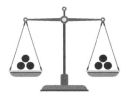

Use Mental   Awareness
Shortcuts   of Bias

BALANCE

Use of mental shortcuts
+ Constant reflection to
avoid bias traps

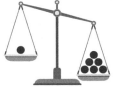

Use Mental   Awareness
Shortcuts   of Bias

NO BALANCE

Not enough use of mental shortcuts
leads to overwhelm, lack of decision
making, mental stress

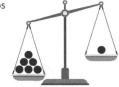

Use Mental   Awareness
Shortcuts   of Bias

NO BALANCE

Not enough awareness of bias,
mistakes will be made

To summarise, most problems result from the third graphic above, where all staff within the NHS are running on Mental Shortcuts and not doing enough reflecting for Bias Traps. This compounds and gets worse, and the underlying pressure in the system becomes more significant – which, as we all know, is extreme. This concept is called "Reciprocal Narrowing" by academics.[95] This research was done around addiction, but the principles are universal, i.e. the more overwhelming the world becomes, the more you narrow it down. Narrow in the sense of rejecting information. This rejection of crucial information could be in the form of taking drugs to numb you to the world (in the case of addiction) or relying too much on mental shortcuts that turn out to be inappropriate Bias (in the case of a nurse).

The result is that you make poor decisions because you do not consider enough relevant information. These poor decisions create a vicious downward spiral of more overwhelm and pressure, narrowing, and constant decline... if you make a mistake on the ward, the pressure builds even more. You become even less able to receive relevant information.

Another early example at the start of this downward spiral could be: You are feeling overwhelmed, so you don't notice your colleagues walking by in the corridor, and you don't say 'Hi'. They think you have 'blanked them', but you are simply dealing with too much to behave in your usual friendly manner. Behaviour like this can impact many levels.

Does this sound familiar in terms of NHS systems?[96] It's natural and understandable – this is a classic response to how humans respond to stress and overwhelm. It's normal; we should not blame people and set certain groups (e.g. managers) up as "the bad guys" – this is a universal situation for everyone.

To make this language more accessible, I use the term **"Mental Narrowing"** to represent this reciprocal narrowing concept.

Please note that the opposite can and does occur, and this is the focus of this entire book: Solutions delivered through appropriate "Mental Openings". You reflect and become aware of Bias. You collect the right

---

95   https://deepfix.substack.com/p/addiction-is-between-you-and-the#:~:text=In%20 cognitive%20science%2C%20reciprocal%20narrowing,object%2C%20we%20are%20after.
96   If not, re-read section 1 of this book.

balance of information, make better decisions, improve results, and reduce stress and overwhelm![97]

Mental Narrowing:

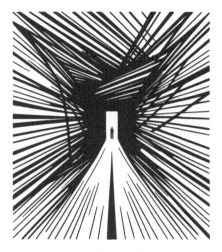

Mental Opening:

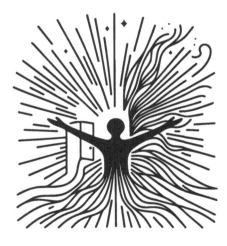

---

97 NB Professor John Seddon refers to "failure demand" in his work (see his book Freedom from Command and Control), and I believe that this concept is very similar to my concept of "problems generated through excessive mental narrowing".

The art of all this is to strike the optimal balance to get as close to the truth as possible, to find the best solution and become "Fit to Care".

It is often easier to spot bias in other people. Look for instances where people are causing problems due to excessive "mental narrowing". The more you do this, the easier it will become to spot when you fall into these bias traps.

Make notes of colleague examples below:

6.4   Thinking fast when you need to think slow![98]

Two more critical Bias examples to pay particular attention to:

1. The difference between causation and correlation. Think of a very large wedding. Statistically, you will likely have a longer marriage if you have a big wedding. However, you'd be silly if you were very poor, spending all your money and getting loans to host such a wedding in the belief that that will make you have a longer marriage.

There is a connection, but it's just a correlation rather than a causation.

The causation factors are as follows: i) If you've an extensive base of family and friends, you will likely have a more solid connection and support network to help you through that marriage. And ii) If you can afford a very large wedding, you have wealth to support you through that long marriage. They're the likely causation factors.

However, the big wedding is just a correlation; the many bottles of champagne will not directly contribute to the marriage's longevity.

2. A second example – thinking too fast when you need more consideration. For example:

You're told that a lily pad has just been introduced to a pond and that it will double in size and surface area daily. On day 20, the pond is finally wholly covered in lily pads.

So, the question is, what day was the pond half covered in lily pads?

Many people will say an instant gut reaction (Mental Shortcut), thinking it was half the time so that it would have been day 10. But that's jumping to conclusions using Mental Shortcuts in the wrong context. You made an error because it's not day 10; it's day 19. It goes from half full on day 19 to completely covered on day 20.

---

98   Thinking, Fast and Slow by Daniel Kahneman (Kahneman, D. (2011). Thinking, Fast and Slow. New York, NY: Farrar, Straus and Giroux.)

Reflection is the key.

 This also ties in with my favourite quote from Socrates: "All I know is that I know nothing." Constantly think – are my thinking and Mental Shortcuts "valuable", or am I Biased because my mental shortcut is inappropriate? (Wrong time, wrong place, wrong context?)

Where can these concepts apply?

The simple answer is EVERYWHERE!

A simplified example: the Blood Pressure you have just taken is high, and it's possible to jump to a Mental Shortcut of genuine medical issues that take you down a particular set of investigations. However, this patient might be known to be consistently prone to white coat syndrome; their BP would be fine at home.

Reflection! Be more like Socrates; sometimes, **you ask more questions** to reduce errors and misunderstandings.

"Let us never consider ourselves finished nurses... we must be learning all of our lives." **Florence Nightingale**

Together for Tomorrow: Pioneering a New Era for the NHS

Chapter 7

Attention to the Wrong Things

7.1 "Pinpointing" or "what's important to you".

How do you decide what's important and what isn't?

The functionality of our brain relating to this "importance" or "salience" stems from hundreds of thousands of years ago when our ancestors were genuinely terrified of animals coming over the hill to eat us. So, in this example, we're afraid of something, and our attention very quickly narrows down to focus everything we have on the attacking beast or running away from it. The academics call this "hyperbolic discounting" because we no longer smell the flowers or listen to bird songs – we only recognise the lion – everything else has been "discounted" away. This is evolutionarily sensible and appropriate as it gives us the best chance at survival.

However, this same brain functionality doesn't only happen when you are attacked! The same mental mechanisms also apply to us *when we want something*.

So, you might recall studies from when you were a child and hearing about various tests where children were offered chocolate and sweets. If they could wait, they'd get even more chocolate or sweets ("Mental Opening" required). And almost invariably, most children couldn't wait and just had to eat the chocolate. The "nowness" of the chocolate becomes overpowering. They can't notice other children or the football game going on. Excessive "Mental Narrowing" has kicked in!

To make the language more accessible, rather than salience or hyperbolic discounting, I call this **"Pinpointing"**.

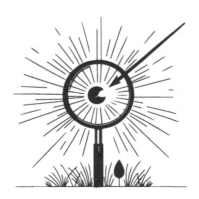

Most of us would feel that, as adults, we use logic to ensure that these Pinpointing Bias Traps don't happen to us. But all too often, we entirely self-delude ourselves ("Bullshit[99]" ourselves), and we do fall into the same traps of Pinpointing and believing in the importance of something NOW, even when it isn't that important or it can even be inappropriate to do so.

 Have you ever looked back on a work decision you made and realised, with the benefit of hindsight, that it was completely the wrong issue? For example, are you so focused on the importance of the checklist and 38.0 degrees that you miss all the other relevant factors?

Another example would be chocolate cake. I love chocolate cake. (There's a lot of chocolate in this chapter!) I could tell myself, "It's only one piece of chocolate cake".

So, I'm bringing that small piece of logic into play, and that alone could justify my decision to eat that chocolate because I'm being overpowered by the "nowness" of it and my desire for it.

This **small** piece of logic (it's only one piece of the jigsaw) is so powerful that it deludes us when we Pinpoint it. However, this data is too narrow to make an appropriate decision; excessive Mental Narrowing is at play.

What we need to do is apply appropriate "Mental Opening". For example, we know that we use this line on ourselves all too often, so we eat the cake daily. We then realise that this results in weight gain and damage to our gut microbiome, which increases our chances of long-term conditions and reduces our ability to care for our loved ones...

A more complete analysis of the relevant data (through Mental Opening) reduces chocolate's impact and "nowness". Then, you can act sensibly, i.e. only eat chocolate in moderation.

You can see how easy it is to fall into this Bias trap, and the same effect happens with cigarettes, alcohol, and all sorts of things. Another work example would be meetings:

---

99 On Bullshit by Harry G. Frankfurt (Frankfurt, H. G. (2005). On Bullshit. Princeton, NJ: Princeton University Press.)

Pinpointing / narrow logic (used to delude ourselves): "We always meet on Tuesday afternoons with my team. It's good to get everyone together." However, through Mental Opening and more significant analysis, you realise that not everyone is getting something out of it. Some members might as well be sitting under the table for the level of input they are giving. It might even be a completely wrong type of meeting (covered in chapter 11).

So, we easily and often delude ourselves into accepting dysfunction, sometimes to avoid conflict. But if we let these delusions build up, the number of problems generated becomes vast.

Professor John Seddon believes that the waste associated with this kind of scenario, in many different forms (he calls failure demand), can impact the NHS's productivity by as much as 80%[100]. I have discovered that NHS managers don't like the term "Failure Demand", so my term is **"Workaround and Rework Time"** (WRT).

 Takeaways To Remember:

- Pinpointing and overwhelming "Nowness" happen all the time. 1) It can be critical to save your life in times of danger, but 2) it can also result in excessive mental narrowing, leading to bias, poor decisions, poor results, and greater overwhelm.
- This almost always results in Workaround and Rework Time (WRT), more work for everyone, and poor patient care/outcomes.
- Always reflect and be mindful of when this could happen to you.

7.2 An NHS personal example of jumping into an incorrect Mental Shortcut

(This is a summary of events as there are too many clinical interactions to document.)

---

100   In command-and-control service organisations, failure demand is astonishingly high, routinely running at 40 – 60% of total customer demand. However, in some sectors, including health and social care, it can escalate to as high as 80% or more, presenting a significant burden on capacity and cost. https://beyondcommandandcontrol.com/

In August 2021, I had a bad cough for at least a month. I had a severe nasal drip the whole time, too. The GP, probably overwhelmed, issued antibiotics. When they did not work, he referred me for a chest X-ray. The X-ray was inconclusive, and so I was put onto a COPD pathway. The waitlist was significant, and I was struggling for about nine months before a different GP escalated my case. I then had all the COPD tests – which confirmed that I did not have COPD.

Then, many appointments later, it was felt that I could have sinusitis. Steroids, another long wait, and more escalation resulted in no polyps or signs of sinus problems.

I then started to feel chest pains and had trouble with my running (a real passion of mine). Then, heart tests, etc.

It was only through a random podcast that I heard (from a Canadian gastroenterologist) that I had a eureka moment – he was explaining GERD and all the symptoms, and I realised – that's me! (NB reflux symptoms can be hardly noticeable and still cause these problems.)

I have subsequently reduced alcohol, caffeine and chocolate, and the transformation has been remarkable.

To summarise.

I believe most GPs I saw were overwhelmed with too many daily appointments. Inevitably, this results in a high chance that they will undergo excessive Mental Narrowing and will jump to a Mental Shortcut too quickly, e.g. COPD pathway. (NB, could this also have been influenced by inappropriate QOF targets?) Ten more minutes of a robust evaluation (Mental Opening) would have revealed that I am a non-smoker and exercise a lot, etc. Not only could I have avoided two inappropriate pathways and dozens of NHS interactions, but also, more than 16 months of poor and troublesome health.[101]

---

101 This is another example of what Professor John Seddon calls "Failure Demand" and I call Workaround and Rework Time (WRT)

7.3   Fixed Mental Shortcuts

A fixed Mental Shortcut is when you have used a Mental Shortcut (often successfully over a long period) to such a degree that you can't see another way – your view and opinion have become "fixed". So even when this mental shortcut causes bias and problems, you still can't see how to "Break the frame" to make a new, more appropriate mental shortcut to "fit" the new situation.

The following illustration is a fantastic insight into this phenomenon:

Draw nine dots[102] like this.

Illustration 1

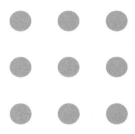

Simple challenge: we need four straight lines to cross all the dots. The lines must be straight. They must cross all the dots; you can do this without taking your pen off the paper.

Okay, so try this now. Sixty seconds to see how you get on. I want to make it clear that this is solvable. So, hopefully, you **believe** you can do it based on that statement. But what you'll find as you start to run through this exercise is that belief doesn't help you. You might have noticed many gurus and online self-help people saying, "Just believe", and everything will be fine. But that, indeed, in this example, is nonsense. Belief doesn't help.

Take a few minutes to try to reach the solution...

Take as much time as you need before turning the page for the solution.

---

102 The 9 dot problem first appeared in a form resembling today's version in an interview with Sam Loyd in The Strand Magazine in 1907

7.4   Solution / Insight (9 dots):

Illustration 2

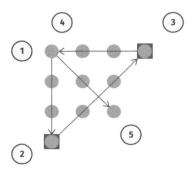

So, the solution is you start at one of the corners (point 1), and you go down, and you **imagine** a fourth dot (point 2), which then enables you to go up diagonally; it's another straight line through those two dots to another **imaginary fourth dot** (point 3), across to the start (point 4) and then back down through to point 5. So, you've got four straight lines in one movement.

Now, I just mentioned there's nothing to do with belief, which is correct. It's also nothing to do with effort. What you did, or many people do, is that they create a constraint that isn't there. See illustration three below. This challenge is difficult for 99% of people (who see it for the first time) because of the old, historic Mental Shortcuts they've created over the years. As children draw by numbers and join the dots, they've created a constraint, a rule of thumb/Mental Shortcut: "Don't go outside the dots (represented by the square – Illustration 3). The square becomes a sort of blindfold you can't see beyond, no matter how hard you try. It doesn't matter what your belief systems are with this. **You can't see what you can't see.**

Illustration 3 – Creating a Constraint (a box) that isn't there:

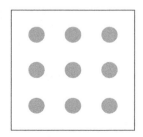

This is a great example of understanding that constraints often exist within your head, and you are unaware of them! These pre-built Mental Shortcuts within you are so powerful that they can have both positive and negative impacts on your daily life.

Therefore, we must be constantly mindful of this. We must build **Mental Openness and curiosity into our daily lives to "break these frames" and boxes in our minds;** to reduce Bias/mistakes and optimise our decision-making and solution-finding skills.

Understanding this must be the start. Only then can you have the awareness and the ability to improve.

Exercise this week at work:

Try to be conscious of where you might be closing things down (because you think there could be no other way).

Notes:

7.5   A Lack of Constraint Analysis

Galileo first formulated the Law of Inertia, which states that if a body is at rest or moving at a constant speed in a straight line, it will remain so unless or **until another force acts upon it**.

The "other force" is particularly relevant for us to remember. Often, our Mental Shortcuts **assume** that our decisions and actions will move us forward and our momentum will carry us onward without a glitch. However, Mental Shortcuts can be too narrow and fail to acknowledge these "other forces" that will slow or derail our initiatives.

For Example:

For example, the doctor had administered an accurate diagnosis and prescription, but there was a failure to consider the "other forces". This patient might have dementia and is failing to remember to take the medication at the right time and the correct dose. In this scenario, an **additional initiative** / Mental Shortcut will have to be applied, e.g. a medication dispenser that is automated to alarm at the correct times of the day and is replenished by the district nurse once a week. Mental Shortcut process 1 (prescription), although accurate, is not delivering outcomes without the proper Mental Opening to consider the "other factor" of compliance, which in turn triggers Mental Shortcut process 2 (electronic dispenser), which means the difference between success and failure of the desired outcomes.

We must be constantly aware and mindful that we are sufficiently Mentally Open to avoid Bias Traps. You can see in this example that a failure of Mental Opening to anticipate the constraint will result in the prescription not working and the patient becoming ill/worse, and this, in turn, will result in more NHS resources and stress on the healthcare system.[103]

7.6   *Work Reflection:*

It's often easier to spot BIAS in other people. Look for instances where people are using mental shortcuts and you know that they are missing important information… e.g. you know something that they don't but they refuse to listen, i.e. their mental shortcut is creating a "fixed frame" that they can't / do not want to break / change.

---

103   This is a good example of what Professor John Seddon calls "Failure demand" and I call Workaround and Rework Time (WRT)

Make notes of these examples below:

BONUS:

Educate a work colleague on SECTION 3 of this book and ask them to actively look for your bias in action. Get them to actively look for your fixed frames / Mental Shortcuts. (only when you are aware, can you break the frame for a more appropriate one.)

NB working as a team – turn this into a game. The more biases that you spot (and you both agree to them being biases) the more points you score – who gets the most points at the end of the week?

*"Nursing is one of the Fine Arts:
I had almost said, the finest of Fine Arts."*
Florence Nightingale

Together for Tomorrow: Pioneering a New Era for the NHS

Chapter 8

Knowledge Gaps and Wisdom

Now that we have the fundamental understanding and language, we can directly link to our work experiences in the NHS. This is where it gets very insightful...

Have you ever thought, **"Why are managers implementing this? They have no idea..."**

As you are probably aware now, after the previous two chapters, the reason for this is Mental Narrowing, i.e. the managers making the decisions are misusing Mental Shortcuts.

8.1 Case Study

A recent example from an NHS Programme (I will not get too specific for reasons of information governance).

There was a significant problem within a particular pathway. One of the big four consultancies was commissioned, and they produced a glossy report and business case. The report was very compelling:

Invest in this technology and implementation (significant investment £s), and the benefits will be:

- improved management information
- improved staff utilisation
- improved consumables usage and commissioning
- better treatment of patients
- reduced bed days in hospitals

Etc.

On paper, it was a no-brainer decision and investment.

My role was to figure out why this initiative wasn't working...

8.2 The 4Ps / 4Ks

To help answer this, I would first like to introduce the work of Professor John Vervaeke (he of the chess example), as this will aid the explanation.

Vervaeke, in his epic 50-hour lecture series "Awakening from the Meaning Crisis"[104], explains, for true knowledge and wisdom, we must have four levels of knowledge – ALL FOUR:

1. **Propositional (Academic logic)**
2. **Procedural (Skills)**
3. **Perspectival (Situational awareness)**
4. **Participatory (Taking part)**

---

104 Intro https://www.youtube.com/ watch?v=ncd6q9uIEdw&list=PLND1JCRq8Vuh3f0P5qjrSdb5eC1ZfZwWJ Detail https://www. youtube.com/watch?v=DxLogRVfBv8

Many people find the language of the 4Ps difficult to grasp and so from now onwards I will refer to the 4Ks instead: Academic Knowledge / Skill Knowledge / Viewpoint Knowledge / Doing Knowledge (ASVD).

Academic Knowledge refers to the knowledge about facts or 'truths'. It's what we often consider as traditional knowledge or information that can be stated explicitly in words or numbers. While essential, relying solely on Academic knowledge is insufficient, as it **doesn't provide the full depth of understanding.**

Skills Knowledge is about skills and practices and **how to do things**. It is developed through practice and enables us to navigate the world effectively and adapt to new challenges.

Viewpoint Knowledge involves seeing the world from a particular viewpoint or context, including the subjective experience of being in a situation. It gives us alternative insights into the world, allowing for **empathy and a deeper understanding**. For example, a nurse and doctor could look at the same patient scenario differently.

Doing Knowledge is the most profound, involving a co-creative relationship between the individual and the world. It's about being part of something larger than oneself and **deeply engaging with practices**, communities, and environments that shape our identity and understanding.

Integrating these 4Ks facilitates wisdom by ensuring a holistic approach to understanding. Wisdom emerges not just from knowing facts (Academic) but from experiencing the world (Viewpoint), engaging with it (Skills), and participating in its ongoing unfolding (Doing). This comprehensive engagement with the world cultivates an adaptive, flexible, and deep understanding essential for navigating the complexities of the NHS with insight and compassion. **Nurses are vital in going beyond the Academic to unlock the additional 3Ks!**

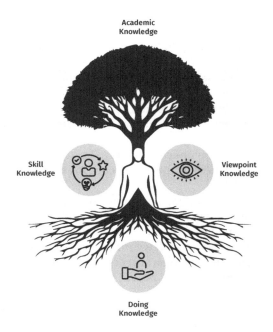

Academic Knowledge

Skill Knowledge

Viewpoint Knowledge

Doing Knowledge

When you become mindful of this, you realise (and see it all the time) that managers (removed from the direct care) making decisions often only operate at one level of knowledge – Academic Knowledge (i.e. a form of Mental Narrowing). At this level of knowledge, they can see 1 + 1 = 2 (in the case above – how logical and appealing the Management Consultant's business case was); however, they are simply missing much of the other three levels of knowledge, which MUST be part of the analysis if you are to manage a successful project.

Direct care staff, especially nurses, are a gold mine of information when it comes to:

2 Skills knowledge, e.g. nurses have this knowledge to be able to implement the initiative (or not).

3 Viewpoint knowledge, e.g. understanding the initiative from their specific role and viewpoint (and they are closest to the patient and their perspectives, too).

4 Doing knowledge, e.g. it's only when you actually "do it" that you deeply understand it.

In this example, it was clear from interviewing nurses that only Academic knowledge had been meaningfully applied to the business case.

Feedback from the nurses to illustrate these "Gaps" included:

- The technology is not easy to use.
- The lighting within patients' houses is often too poor to get an acceptable image.
- Because of XYZ, I don't have the time to be able to see the patient and collect the data that "they" expect us to collect, etc.

The list of these issues was long, and after review, you can see that "it's a no-brainer that this initiative WON'T WORK – is obvious". The business case writers are just operating at the Academic level and have Mentally Narrowed from the other three levels of knowledge. Quite simply, this mistake is the difference between success and failure and one of the primary reasons for writing this book.

NB I was also impressed with the nurses (some very junior) who had LOTS OF SOLUTIONS but felt hamstrung in sharing and implementing these ideas.

This Mental Narrowing of not considering the other three levels of knowledge is partly cultural (that we will explore further later in the book) and partly due to overwhelm, which was covered in Chapter 6.

8.3   Other Examples

Look at these high-profile IT infrastructure projects that have not lived up to expectations:

1. Ministry of Defence – secure military network infrastructure project. Initial budget 2.3 billion and the latest estimate £7.1 billion

2. NHS National IT Programme – this project that cost over £10 billion was abandoned in September 2013

3. Magistrates Libre System – This project was initially budgeted for £146m. Still, after a series of substantial price increases, the contract had to be renegotiated with another supplier, generating significant losses for the taxpayer.

Do you think that this Pinpointing on Academic knowledge business cases could be endemic within the public sector? I do... and it's not only IT projects; think back to the Poll Tax!

I believe that these problems are universal and occur in every organisation. However, the NHS is so overwhelmed, which results in excessive Mental Narrowing – it's predictable and inevitable, leading to further Workaround and Rework stress in the system.

"For the sick it is important to have the best." **Florence Nightingale**

Together for Tomorrow: Pioneering a New Era for the NHS

Chapter 9

Insights To Help with Our Solutions

Insights To Help with Our Solutions Introduction

In chapter 6, we covered "Overwhelm" and how the human brain is bombarded with colossal amounts of information daily (remember the Chess Board example with more potential legal moves that there are particles in the universe).

We then understood why it's essential for the human brain to "spot patterns" in the mass of information and create "Mental Shortcuts" so that we can get through the day practically without a mental breakdown. These Mental Shortcuts can be represented as world views/frames/boxes.

By understanding these Mental shortcuts/frames, we can see how the brain can rely on them too heavily and in inappropriate situations (wrong place, wrong time, wrong context), resulting in Bias, poor decisions, and poor outcomes.

For example, if you create a mental frame that **"patient X is very needy and asks for a lot of attention unnecessarily"**, which might be useful when it comes to adjusting bed sheets (20 times per day[105]), but that frame would be wholly inappropriate when the same patient says, "I am in a lot of pain". Relevant frames in some situations can be irrelevant and wrong in different settings and scenarios; i.e. it might be appropriate to ignore the bed sheet adjustment occasionally, but not to fall into the same mental frame of discounting when the patient is in pain.

Let's link this to the 4Ks

Picture each form of knowledge (Academic/Skills/Viewpoint/Doing) as a Mental Shortcut.

The square represents Academic; Triangle, Skills; Circle, Viewpoint; and Star, Doing.

All these frames and world views have value, but in isolation, they cannot generate the wisdom required for the "FIT", i.e. the optimal[106] decisions/outcomes.

---

105 For aesthetic reasons, not related to bed sore management.

106 In the sense of the best we can achieve, given the constraints we are dealing with, we will never achieve perfection.

Where the predominant worldview/frame is the academic square, and you build an initiative just on this alone, it will always be far from efficient and effective, as we saw from examples in the previous chapter. Similarly, if a direct care worker with lots of knowledge of the other 3Ks doesn't understand the Academic knowledge of business case processes, cash flow, etc., then that initiative is likely to fall short, too.

All four areas of knowledge (including authentic teamwork to glean these insights) are required for wisdom, which is what we strive for. We must work with colleagues and all relevant stakeholders to have good knowledge in all four areas, can see the golden thread, and generate wisdom.

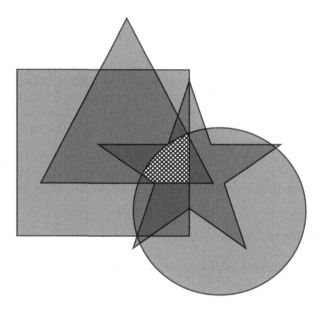

For example, there has been a top-down policy (Academic knowledge) that no infection should be considered if the patient's temperature is under 38 degrees.

But in the actual situation, you have an experienced nurse bringing her 92-year-old father into A&E (with lots of skill knowledge) who has been closely following her father's temperature for that past day. You can see it rising quickly (Viewpoint knowledge). His temperature is now 37.9, the trend is up, and the daughter is concerned about sepsis because of his broken ribs (Doing knowledge). In this scenario, the 4Ks combined generate much more wisdom than the Academic knowledge alone. At the very least, you would ask a colleague for advice if unsure rather than dismiss it because the temperature was not yet 38.0 degrees.

However, as we saw with the nine dots exercise, it's very easy to get trapped into a particular frame (in this case, 38.0 degrees) to such an extent that you can't think about or "see" anything else. This is where you commonly experience the "computer says no" syndrome. Add stress and overwhelm, and you are even more likely to experience these scenarios of inappropriate Mental Narrowing.

Critical thinking and Mental Opening are much easier when you consider the 4Ks rather than just the common Academic Knowledge as the focal point.

9.1 Summary and Solutions Required.

The brain is amazing and can process vast amounts of information very well. However, these insights in Section 3 also remind us to be constantly vigilant for excessive Mental Narrowing (in various forms). Socrates's quote, "All I know is that I know nothing", can remind us to stay mindful and reflective.

 Takeaways To Remember:

1. Sometimes, our Mental Shortcuts are so powerful that we can't see any other way (remember the nine dots challenge).
2. Sometimes, we assume that our Mental Shortcut/solution will have no "other factors" to influence it. This is another form of Mental Narrowing, and without proper constraint analysis, most projects will not deliver great results.
3. Finally, we get to John Vervaeke's work on the 4Ps (which we refer to as the 4Ks) and realise that we can only get to wisdom when we have Mental Openness to all four levels of Academic, Skills, Viewpoints and Doing knowledge. The predominant weakness in most management teams is not engaging sufficiently with direct care staff (particularly nurses) to gain all four levels of knowledge.

Below is an illustration to act as an aide memoir for Section 3 of the book.

Illustration – Aide Memoir

Ultimately, we are aiming for Optimal Mental Balance:

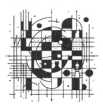

Information Overwhelm

Mental Shortcuts

Bias
(inappropriate Mental Shortcut – wrong time / place /context)

Pinpointing
(Great in danger. But Problematic Mental Narrowing with desires).

Fixed Mental Shortcuts
(just can't see another way, stuck within the box)

Lack of Constraint Analysis
(assuming no "other forces will influence")

Knowledge Gaps (4Ps)
(Propositional, Procedural, Perspectival, Participatory)

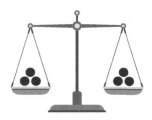

Use Mental   Awareness
Shortcuts   of Bias

BALANCE

Use of mental shortcuts
+ Constant reflection to
avoid bias traps

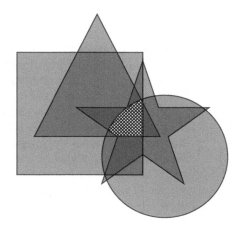

9.2   Insights to Practical Next Steps.

From Section 3 of the book, we have made a case for:

a. Being aware of when you might have fallen into an excessive Mental Narrowing situation.
b. Be aware of when you might be Pinpointing inappropriately.
c. Being aware of when you might have a Fixed Mental Shortcut to the point where you can't see that you are causing problems.
d. We must make a conscious effort to open our minds to consider all the relevant "other forces" and ensure that constraints do not derail our work.

The consistent underlying theme is that we must be **mindful** of when we excessively use Mental Shortcuts (Mental Narrowing).

 Takeaways To Remember:

- Take time to STOP and reflect – culturally, this must be an acceptable part of the job (and it saves time and resources in the long run, as it reduces Workarounds and Rework).
- Work together in teams, as it's often easier to see other people's bias traps than to see your own (especially at the start of this process). To achieve this teamwork, we must first build trust within the team.

  – Utilise tools and techniques to "Break Mental Shortcuts" when you can't see a way out; especially Insight-Genie[107] (see voucher at the end of the book).

  These techniques help us "break the frame" to consider all 4Ks, allowing us to create new, more appropriate Mental Shortcuts and solutions.

---

107 www.fittocare.co.uk/insight-genie (Other tools and techniques that we use that you will also explore if you join our courses are: – Think in the third person, – View from Above, – The Naked Truth, – Metaphors, – Mind Maps)

John Vervaeke's Awakening from the Meaning Crisis concludes that life is all about "Fitting" to our environments and purpose, and that's what Optimal Mental Balance enables us to work towards.

 Insight

> Now you can see a deeper meaning to the title of this book, **"Fit** To Care". This is all about optimising your life, purpose, and happiness. Improving patient outcomes will be a significant part of this, but you can see now that there is much more to this journey.

This "Fitting to the environment" is about achieving the best results, and it applies to individuals as well as organisations.

From an individual perspective, how you relate to everyone around you (at home and work) is critical. You will need the right Mental Balance to achieve your best interactions.

From an organisational perspective, you need the right Mental Balance from the whole organisation so that every stakeholder is marching to the same tune to achieve the same goals.

9.3   So, what are the Goals?

Now we can optimise our Mental Balance to achieve more tremendous success, what are we aiming to achieve?

Viktor Frankl, a psychologist who survived five concentration camps of the Nazi holocaust, was well qualified to study Meaning and "What is life all for?" and he concluded that three core elements deliver meaning and happiness (even under Nazi brutality).[108]

1 Creativity. Your gifts to the world. Work that utilises your unique skills and talents, e.g. your vocation of caring for people

---

108 If this is a topic that you would like to learn more about, I would highly recommend the book "Viktor Frankl's Logotherapy" by Ann Graber.

2 Experiences. Gifts from the world to you. This could be a family member's unconditional love, gratitude from a patient or a sunset's beauty.

3 Attitude. The purpose you have and how you frame a situation. What is important to you.

John Vervaeke asks, **"What would you like to continue after you're gone?"** This is an excellent way to tie you to your "Attitude" and Meaning/purpose (we will develop this further in section 4).

For Frankl and Vervaeke, happy and productive lives are not linked to fame or fortune!

When we identify our personal and organisational Meaning and purpose, we can utilise our skills and techniques to "Fit" our environments to achieve our purpose and goals optimally; we realise our relevance in the world and feel great in the process.

 Reflection

We are most happy and productive when we are on a journey and working/progressing towards a goal that has Meaning for us. You might have sensed "the flow state"[109] before, where you are in a state of extreme productivity, hardly conscious of what you are doing and what is around you... This state is usual when operating at a high level, and the task is based on something meaningful with a purpose for you. Have you experienced this yet?

If not, I hope this book will be the start of this journey for you.

---

109 Flow: The Psychology of Optimal Experience by Mihaly Csikszentmihalyi

"Wise and humane management of the patient is the best safeguard against infection." **Florence Nightingale**

Together for Tomorrow: Pioneering a New Era for the NHS

Section 4

The Solutions

Solutions Introduction

Sections 1 and 2 evidenced the tension and gap between where we are now and what we need to achieve. Section 3 introduced you to the high-level concepts and developed your ability to recognise errors in thinking and decision-making that will impact you and your team.

In section 4, we aim to facilitate the use of what you have learned. You can now start embedding the Fit to Care Methodology and the 4 As, Aspirations, Actions, Anchors, and Autopilot (which will be explained) into everything that you do in terms of practical development and implementation.

The illustration below summarises the complete Fit To Care System. It's the vehicle that takes us from current Problems to the Payoff of you being "Fit" and a lot happier working for the NHS and serving patients as you want to.

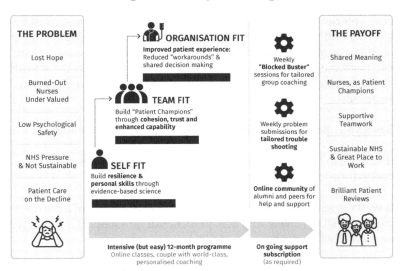

The Fit to Care System
3 Training and Development Programmes

Implementing the 5 Foundations for Every Initiative

| Meaning | Attitude | Skills | Guidelines | Systems |

Self Fit, is all about looking after yourself. If you are not fit, your family and patients will suffer, so this must be the starting point. This first course is about learning the essential skills, techniques, and shared language you can use in the following two courses.

Team Fit is all about team norms, how you can support one another and make quick wins in your everyday environment to make your working days easier and leave at the end of the day with a smile and purpose in your step.

Organisation / Patient Fit can then draw upon your new skills/ teamwork and support you in making more radical system thinking design changes to your working systems to reduce your workloads and improve patient care.

It is worth noting that most projects associated with change and improvement attempt to start at level 3 (Organisation Fit) and then wonder why it rarely makes any impact.

We must start with YOU as an individual.

Before you can get the most out of life at home and work, you must be physically and mentally "fit". Utilising our "Fit to Care" methodology will seamlessly apply evidence-based science and systems thinking to your life to overcome the roadblocks that get in your way. Utilise these skills to improve your career prospects and make a difference to those you care about.

What's your baseline starting position – how "Fit" are you?

The American Psychiatric Association introduced the generalised anxiety disorder (GAD) tool in 1980.

It is well recognised within the NHS as a good barometer of a person's anxiety and stress levels, and this, in turn, can be a helpful insight into how mentally fit you are.

Dr Robert Sapolsky[110] explores how **prolonged stress** can lead to severe physical and mental health issues, drawing on a wealth of scientific research to explain the mechanisms behind stress-related diseases in humans.

---

110 Sapolsky, R. M. (2004). Why Zebras Don't Get Ulcers. New York: St. Martin's Press.

The impact of Stress:

Activates the Fight-or-Flight Response: Stress triggers the body's primal fight-or-flight response, preparing us to confront or escape danger. This involves a surge in adrenaline and cortisol, increasing heart rate, blood pressure, and energy supplies.

Impacts on Mental Health: Chronic stress can lead to mental health issues such as depression, anxiety, and mood disorders. It affects neurotransmitter levels, including serotonin and dopamine, contributing to feelings of sadness and hopelessness.

Affects Immune Function: Prolonged stress suppresses the immune system, making us more susceptible to infections and illnesses. It can also slow down the healing process and exacerbate autoimmune diseases.

Increases Risk of Heart Disease: Stress increases inflammation in the body, a risk factor for heart disease. It can lead to higher cholesterol levels, arterial damage, and hypertension.

Contributes to Weight Gain: High levels of cortisol associated with stress can lead to overeating and weight gain. Stress-induced cravings often involve high-fat, sugary foods, contributing to obesity.

Impairs Memory and Concentration: Chronic stress can damage the hippocampus, the part of the brain responsible for memory and learning, leading to difficulties in concentration and memory recall.

Disrupts Sleep: Stress can cause insomnia and disrupt sleep patterns, leading to fatigue, decreased productivity, and further stress.

Affects Digestive System: Stress can lead to gastrointestinal issues, such as irritable bowel syndrome (IBS), ulcers, and indigestion, due to altered digestive functioning.

Influences Behaviour: It can lead to unhealthy coping mechanisms, such as alcohol or drug abuse, social withdrawal, and aggression.

Reduces Job Satisfaction and Performance: Stress can diminish concentration, decision-making ability, and overall job satisfaction in the workplace, impacting performance and relationships with colleagues.

Sapolsky's research underscores the need for stress management interventions in professional settings, especially in high-stress environments like healthcare, to support mental and physical health. We must take this seriously!

Consider these questions below.[111] Reflect on the last two weeks and score yourself as honestly as possible. Remember to take the test after implementing the initiatives in the book to see how you are improving.

GAD Questions to reflect upon Over the last 2 weeks, how often have you been bothered by...	Definintions and Scores			
	Not at all	Several days	Over half days	Nearly every day
Feeling nervous, anxious, or on edge?	0	1	2	3
Not being able to stop of control worrying?	0	1	2	3
Worrying too much about different things?	0	1	2	3
Trouble relaxing?	0	1	2	3
Being so restless that it's hard to sit still?	0	1	2	3
Becoming easily annoyed or irritable?	0	1	2	3
Feeling afraid as if something awful might happen?	0	1	2	3

111 Generalized Anxiety Disorder (GAD) American Psychiatric Association. (2013). Diagnostic and Statistical Manual of Mental Disorders (5th ed.). Washington, DC: Author.

Score Results

Normal (0-4)	No change necessary.
Mild Anxiety (5-9)	Consider changes to your life.
Moderate Anxiety (10-14)	Don't ignore this level of anxiety. You could have Genralised Anxiety Disorder (GAD) and should see your GP.
Severe Anxiety (15+)	Do something about this. Arrange a GP appointment as a priority.

Source: Spitzer RL, Kroenke K, Williams JBW, Lowe B. A brief measure for assessing generalized anxiety disorder. Arch Inern Med. 2006;166:1092-1097

Write your current score in the book below – do it now and date it. Compare it again after you have completed the book and the exercises, to track your progress!

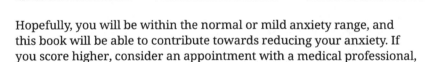

Hopefully, you will be within the normal or mild anxiety range, and this book will be able to contribute towards reducing your anxiety. If you score higher, consider an appointment with a medical professional, follow this book, and always consider joining our courses at www. FitToCare.co.uk

If you would like your team members to take this review - they can do online with this link https://www.fittocare.co.uk/scorecard

You're busy – we get it!

We understand how busy you are, so this book has been designed to be PRACTICAL and HIGH IMPACT above all else. We know you don't have time to waste!

The Fit to Care Methodology

The illustration below summarises the "getting stuff done/getting change to happen" magic within our practical implementation systems. Section 4 of the book will incorporate these elements.

Practical Implementation

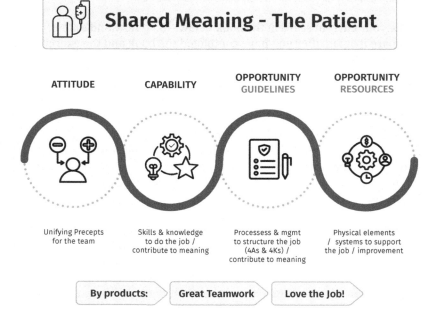

Chapter 10

Self Fit

This Chapter is about YOU and is the first of the three Fit To Care programmes!

You don't need to know how an engine works to be able to drive a car. Similarly, you don't need to know much about Cognitive Science and Behavioural Science to get massive value from this chapter, so we will keep it as short as possible.

Just follow the system and enjoy the process – this programme is intentionally PRACTICAL rather than academic; the best way to learn is through doing!

Please don't just look at the exercises as something to read; **YOU HAVE TO DO THEM,** i.e. physically, grab a pen and paper and think these exercises through. As you go through the chapter, write your notes on this Checklist. You can write into this page of the book or print off from the online Resources www.FitToCare.co.uk/fittocareresources

Self Fit Checklist

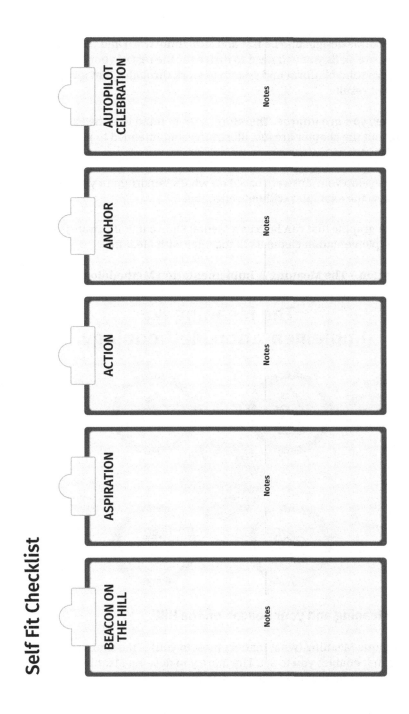

BEACON ON THE HILL

Notes

ASPIRATION

Notes

ACTION

Notes

ANCHOR

Notes

AUTOPILOT CELEBRATION

Notes

The chapter is designed to be fast and straightforward and teaches you the core skills you will need to thrive for the rest of your life. It provides a solid platform and system to work through – that gives consistent results.

However, you are unique. Therefore, keep in mind that the examples throughout the chapter are just illustrative and intended to provide a guide for you.

Please develop your answers based on what's important to you; don't just follow the examples without reflecting.

Here is a graphic that can help as a Mental Shortcut; it illustrates how these implementation elements fit together with Meaning:

Illustration – The Meaning & Implementation Methodology

The Meaning & Implementation Methodology

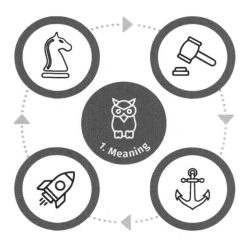

2. Aspiration

Connect Aspirations to what matters, "Meaning" and prioritise the easy wins first.

3. Action

Design the most appropriate Actions that serve your Aspirations.

5. Autopilot

Turn these transforming Actions into Autopilot habits, that make everything so easy.

4. Anchor

Design the most appropriate Anchors that guarantee your Actions.

1. Meaning

10.1   Meaning and your Beacon on the Hill

Your unique Meaning (what matters most to you) is the source of your energy that enables you to act. The more you develop Meaning, the fitter you become, and the more you can achieve.

The method / Mental Shortcut we use to enable you to quickly unlock and understand what's important to you as a unique individual is the following exercise – which is crucial (you will see how it all ties together later in the book).

The "What's important?" exercise:

Professor John Vervaeke[112] asks two profound questions when it comes to meaning and importance:

Q1. "What do you want to exist after you're gone?"

Q2. "What are you currently doing to contribute to these things?"

Most people feel reoriented after the first question and start to doubt what they spend all their time and effort on. The second question often consolidates this feeling of "wrong focus" because they feel that they are not contributing enough to those things that matter.

Remember that these answers can only ever be unique to you, but an illustration to question 1 might be:

Answer 1

"I would really want my partner or children to thrive and prosper if I no longer existed."

OR

"I really want the planet to be sustainable after I'm gone."

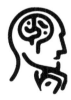 **Please reflect** on this and then write down your unique answers to this question; we call these answers your "Beacons on the Hill" (there can be more than one). Write these on your Self Fit Checklist that you recently saw/printed off. Keep this checklist visible (as well as in your mind) as you work through this book.

Now, onto Question 2… Based on your life right now (before completing this book), how good are your contributions to your Beacon(s) on the

---

112 Professor of Cognitive Science at Toronto University

Hill? Mark yourself out of 10. (You might find that you are exhausted and have little time or energy to contribute to the things that matter to you?)

Please write these answers down, too. By the end of the course, you will see how the skills you develop will enable you to contribute much better to the essential things. As a result, you will have more meaning in your life and feel "fitter" and happier too.

Please do not move forward until you have seriously contemplated this section adequately and written out both your Beacons on the Hill and the strength of your contributions to them.

Some people might find this exercise problematic. If you need to, take your time and sleep on it.

Your personal "Beacon(s) on the Hill" will be a significant component of the programme, and you will see how it all ties in later in the book.

10.2 Contemplate the Difficulties You Face and Set "Aspirations"

ASPIRATIONS

Your daily problems are signals that can help you understand the appropriate "Aspirations". These will contribute to your Beacon on the Hill, which you must focus on. Aspirations are marginally less critical than the Beacon on the Hill; **they should support your ability to serve and contribute to the Beacon on The Hill.**

You must make your list, but here are some illustrative examples of Aspirations to manage that will help you to grasp the concepts:

- I need to get more sleep
- I need to do more exercise
- I need to drink less alcohol
- I should spend more time with friends and family
- I need a better diet...etc.

Note these things are currently a barrier to serving your Meaning/purpose. For example, if your sleep is poor and you are constantly exhausted, no matter what your Beacon on the Hill is, you probably will not be in a fit state to serve it.

Let the list flow – don't worry, this will not become overwhelming, as the next step is to focus on a few of these Aspirations that will support a significant improvement in your strength and well-being.

To help with your lists, consider Mindfulness. Mindfulness (a vital tool) is awareness of your thoughts and feelings in the present moment. Observe your thoughts, feelings, and problems without judging them or yourself.

Sit quietly and contemplate for 10 – 15 minutes. List what you instinctively know is causing you harm, stress, or weakening your well-being. When you have a good list, move on to the next page.

10.3 Shortlisting Aspirations (start easy):

Now, looking at your complete list of difficulties and Aspirations to improve, you will shortlist a top three.

In this shortlist process, consider:

    a.   Which ones would make the most impact on your life?
    b.   Which ones would you love to do/get resolved?

Don't overthink this – identify the top three Aspirations (from the previous page) that you would love to change, which will ultimately make you much more resilient and happier and improve your well-being.

Great. Now, we are making progress. We are ready to move on!

Shortlisting your top three is excellent, as you can systematically manage all three Aspirations when ready. However, for this book, we will develop your skills in one area: learn the system, and then there will be no stopping you.

The next step is to prioritise one of your top three. Let's start with the easiest. For this contemplation, you need to consider five possible constraints (think of five fingers):

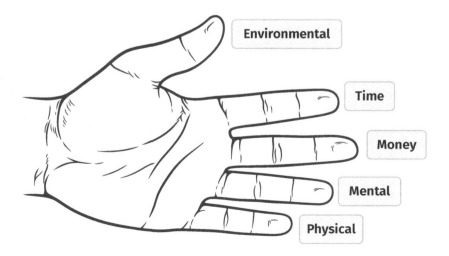

Thinking about your Top Three Aspirations (each in turn), and consider:

1. Time – how long will it take? How precious is your time?
2. Money – how much will this action cost? How much money do you have?
3. Mental Effort – will this be easy for you, or will it be demanding?
4. Physical Effort – will this be easy for you, or will it be demanding?
5. Environmental – what impact will this have on things or people that might be impacted / might hinder your progress?

Hopefully, these criteria will help you **identify one Aspiration for us to work on**: the easiest of your top three shortlisted areas (again, don't overthink this).

For the remainder of this book, we will focus on one Aspiration, e.g. SLEEP. This will, in turn, help your resilience and well-being (and improve your GAD score that we recorded earlier).

NB This example of Sleep as the #1 Aspiration must contribute to your Beacon on the Hill. And it does because a well-rested person will be less stressed, more resilient, and able to take on the world with a passion – including other Aspirations that will contribute directly to the Beacon on the Hill.

When you're happy and keen to develop your #1 Aspiration – update your Self Fit Checklist.

10.4   Recognise your progress!

Well done! You are doing well if you have a Beacon(s) on the Hill and one solid and clear contributory Aspiration. Recognising progress is important – why this is so important will be explained in the following pages. 😊 You are ready for the next challenge!

If, earlier in section 3, you joined forces with a colleague to explore each other's Bias Traps, engage again and share your Beacon(s) on the Hill and priority Aspiration – discuss them. Or you could start to share and talk through with loved ones at home.

10.5 ACTIONS – It's time for the Magic Wand

So now we start our detailed design around supporting the "Aspiration" that you identified earlier (e.g. Improving your sleep) with the most "relevant" Action.

A trick for identifying the most relevant action is to sit quietly and imagine that you have a magic wand and can do any action you want concerning your aspiration.

First, be creative and list all the possibilities (don't worry about the practicalities at this stage).

Illustration example Actions could be (for the example of the sleep Aspiration):

* Fit blackout blinds.
* Fit an air conditioning unit.
* Buy an alarm to set for a prompt bedtime regime.
* Leave your phone in a different room.
* Don't allow the dog in your room at night.
* etc.

Before you move on from this list, could there be any more? Ask a partner or loved one if they can think of anything else (Viewpoint Knowledge). If no one is available, imagine what they would add to the list if they were with you (Breaking frame with a Third-Person analysis, i.e. put yourself in their shoes. What would they think? What would they advise? This can be a great way to break your mental frame).

Feel free to write in the book or download the "Magic Wand Analysis" file on the website[113] to help you with this process.

---

113 www.fittocare.co.uk/fittocareresources

	Magic Wand Actions List	Impact (High 100 Low 0)	How Easy (Easy 100 Hard 0)
1			
2			
3			
4			
5			
6			
7			
8			
9			
10			

Second, consider the **Impacts** of each of these possible Actions.

For example, instantly, you might score blackout blinds as high because you always wake at 4.00 am when it gets light in the summer because of the sun. Alternatively, you might score not allowing the dog into your room as high because he always wakes you three to four times every night without fail.

Remember, these are unique to you – this system allows you to think through quickly and easily. NB When you have developed your skills (after working through the book and some experience), you can run several of these *Aspirations* and corresponding *Actions* simultaneously. But we are just starting things simple so you can learn the ropes.

Thirdly, rank order these Actions (**based on Impacts**) with the highest scores at the top.

10.6   Your #1 Priority Action

From your rank order list of possible Actions based on Impact, it's time to consider "how EASY" each will be accomplished. (Download the file to help if you did not download it in the previous section.)

A high score of 100 means it is VERY EASY. A low score of 0 means you know that it will never happen!

To help with the scoring of these Actions and to help you think through – consider the five fingers again:

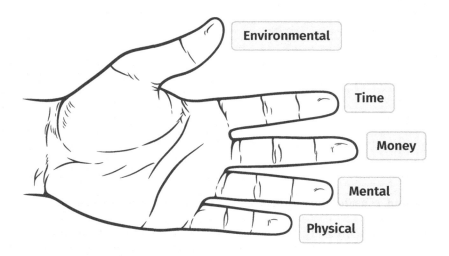

To determine how "easy", consider the impact that each Action has on:

Your TIME

Your MONEY

Your MENTAL EFFORT

Your PHYSICAL EFFORT

The ENVIRONMENT

Analysis of the shortlist:

For example, air conditioning might have scored high on impact, but you know it's impossible, as you have no funds to do it. So, from an "Easy" score perspective, the score would be low.

However, putting your phone in the other room might have scored a high-impact score as you know that you always stay up late watching YouTube shorts (and regret it at 12.30 am). And then, looking at the "Easy" score, that's also high because: 1) It takes no time to do, 2) It costs nothing, 3) Mental effort will be a little challenging, 4) No physical effort, 5) No impact on anyone else in the family.

"BINGO!"

In this illustration, there are very few constraints; this is the #1 Priority Action that we will focus on as it has a high impact and looks relatively easy to do.

This #1 **Action** will be the focus for learning all your skills!

So, illustratively, we now have your #1 Action as "I will put my phone in the other room at 10.30 pm".

But this is only the start... now we get to the exciting parts!

Well Done!

In setting the priority Action, possibly the hardest (potentially most tedious) job is done! Or you might have found it incredibly easy. Either way, don't underestimate this as an achievement.

If you are engaging with a work buddy or family member, update them now on your #1 Action that will support your Aspiration or compare your choices. This, in turn, will contribute to your Beacon on the Hill.

10.7 Create Your Anchor

Now that you have your #1 Action that you will focus on doing regularly, e.g. putting your phone into another room at bedtime, you can start to make a practical difference in your life!

Myth Busting Motivation (Why Anchors are so Important):

Motivation could be compared to "Fun Bobby" from Friends: great to be around when things are good but terrible the day after the party – i.e. Motivation is highly unreliable.

My personal eureka insight was obtained through B.J. Fogg.[114] *We are brainwashed from an early age (a Mental Shortcut) into believing that Motivation is THE KEY FACTOR to behaviour change.* Even the NHS uses the COMB model, too (M stands for Motivation).

Many "Motivational" tools and techniques revolve around Rewards, Incentives and Punishments.[115] However, I believe, although a factor, Motivation is NOT the key, and I believe that evidence of many failed initiatives within the NHS proves me correct.

When you consider behaviour change, we must review these three variables diligently:

1. How Easy is something to do? (Practically)
2. How Hard is it mentally for the person in question to do it? (Cognitive Bias)
3. How motivated is the person to do it? (Existing Mental Shortcuts)

NB Variables 1 and 2 are not the same question reframed.

Just because it's easy to do something practically (1), e.g. click on a link to enter some data, doesn't mean there won't be mental barriers.

(2) Mental difficulty because you have unhelpful Biases, e.g. "I hate computers; face-to-face engagement is the only way to get things done".

The Motivation variable (3) might be "I have no time to do this", and the mental Shortcut driving this could be – "I'm not committed to this project/organisation".

I argue that #1 is the critical variable because if it's EASY (e.g. 1 second to click and 5 seconds to enter your name and click a preference), then the objections from 2 and 3 will be minimal. The more difficult, then the more you are likely to get resistance from both 2 and 3.

We tackle variable 2 by encouraging the 4Ks, creating a culture of breaking frames, and being as conscious of Mental Opening as possible.

---

114 Tiny Habits by BJ Fogg

115 https://www.fittocare.co.uk/insights/blog-post-punish-behaviour

We tackle variable 3 not through dysfunction gimmicks and financial bribes, but through **belonging and shared Meaning.**

All three variables are critical to consider, but the first one, **EASIFICATION** is the most important and needs to be developed with systems thinking and the relevant range of stakeholders to ensure proper 4K wisdom in the design.

 Remember

This is the fundamental equation that we must all ALWAYS remember. *"The harder something is to do; the more frame breaking and motivation is required to achieve it."*

I.e. the core/starting variable that we must focus on is making it easy – so easy, in fact, that it's easier to do the thing you want to get done than not to do it.

Compared to – making something hard and hoping it gets done – when, statistically, it probably won't!

This update in strategic thinking also ties in with **"Hard is often linked to Information Overwhelm and Mental Narrowing"**, which leads to Bias, poor decisions, rework, and general pain...

 Insight

We need to focus on avoiding relying on motivation and willpower. They're unreliable and can even be dysfunctional.

This is also consistent with Professor John Seddon's work. In his NHS experience, system thinking and making the flow of work "easy", frictionless, and focused on the patient journey improved NHS employees' morale and well-being naturally as a by-product of system design and "Easification".

System design and ease of workflow are the drivers, i.e. the cause. Motivation and well-being are the effects. NOT Motivation drives better systems and better morale – because it doesn't; it's a myth.

One key hack for "Easification" to reduce Mental Overwhelm is to piggyback on an already automated habit (our Anchor) that you already do on autopilot. For example, you will already flush the toilet "without thinking". The keywords here are 'without thinking' – literally no cognitive load and no memory required. For example, "I must remember to XYZ" requires mental energy, and we want to minimise this.

We use Anchors because both memory and motivation are unreliable.

For our case study illustration (getting better sleep), we could use "brushing teeth" as our existing relevant "Anchor" to "Trigger" our New #1 Action (taking the phone into the other room).

Note there could be many anchor options, and your choice will be bespoke to you and your particular Action.

Key Considerations when choosing a relevant Anchor are:

1. **Location** – Are you in the right place? You must be able to INSTANTLY move from the Anchor Action (brushing teeth) to the new Action (moving phone).
2. **Time of day** – does the Anchor Action happen at the right time? It must be the right time to allow instantaneous New Action – DO NOT RELY ON MEMORY!
3. **Frequency**–Ideally, you want to match the frequency of the Anchor Action to the Frequency of the New Action – when it does, it will "wire" into your brain even more quickly.

Something you must do – Visualise!

Now that you have identified your relevant Anchor for your #1 Action, the next step is to **visualise** (several times) the existing Anchor and the Trigger to the New Action, e.g. when you put the toothbrush down (visualise the detail) and wipe your hands, that is the trigger for you to take your phone and put it on charge in another room (other than your bedroom) and walk into your bedroom to sleep (or read a little if you prefer) – visualise that whole routine in your mind (are there any stairs on the route, what's the colour of the carpet, is it fiddly to get the charging cable to plug in? Visualise the detail – several times).

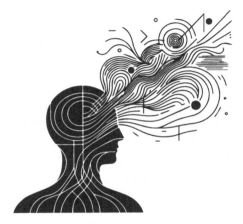

The Anchor is so essential, it's like magic!

Please remember the visualisation, as this is required to "wire in" the trigger moment and to make the whole process super easy.

Only move on when you can vividly picture the Anchor and new Action in your mind!

Note: One often-cited study on this topic is "Habits in Everyday Life: Thought, Emotion, and Action[116]". This study suggested that about **43% of daily behaviours are performed out of habit,** i.e. with no cognitive load – just done on autopilot. Many activities, both at work and home, are done with no or very little cognitive load.

10.8 Feel the Joy! AUTOPILOT

The following essential factor is to "Feel the Joy" of your achievements – DO NOT MISS THIS OUT, as this is another critical piece of the jigsaw!

You might have noticed in the earlier pages that I have been congratulating you along the way… There was a method in my madness!

---

116 by Wendy Wood, Jeffrey M. Quinn, and Deborah A. Kashy, published in 2002. It can be found in the Journal of Personality and Social Psychology.

The feeling of accomplishment is so important because when this happens, we get a dopamine spike in our brain and then these act to "wire a habit" without us even being aware of what we are doing. Our evolutionary systems effectively say, "This is good; do it again".

So, how do we capture this cognitive science into our working system? Easy:

1. Celebrate when the Anchor trigger works. For example, I brush my teeth, and BINGO – my mind tells me (due to the visualisation) to put the phone into the other room. "It worked! Wow, I'm good at this!"
2. Celebrate when you connect the phone in the other room, "I'm doing it, this is brilliant".
3. Celebrate when your head hits the pillow (much earlier than usual): "I am going to feel so much better in the morning – tomorrow is going to be a great day."

Remember, it must be an authentic celebration; don't fake it, as the dopamine won't trigger.

Consider how you usually celebrate when something incredible happens. If you are a football fan and your team scores a last-minute winning goal, do you fist pump the air? Do you shout out "YES"? Or do you do these things in your head? Do whatever is usually authentic to you.

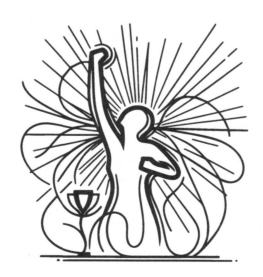

Be Warned:

Sometimes, your mind might say, "Celebrating plugging in a phone – are you serious???? Don't be such an idiot!" (This could be a mental box/ constraint that you placed on yourself many years ago; it doesn't need to be perpetuated. Let's break such inappropriate frames...)

You must NOT fall into this celebration trap. Very simple things (designed well) can lead to transformation change, which is the goal.

In such situations, REFRAME. Pull out your "Beacon(s) on the Hill" that you have written on the Self Fit Checklist (if not already committed to memory).

These celebrations are not silly; they are about something much bigger, e.g. my contribution to my spouse, my children, the environment, etc. (i.e. the Beacons on the Hill list).

In this illustration, getting quality sleep can significantly impact my ability to make much better contributions... you are not just plugging your phone in; you are changing your life...

Now, you are starting to see how the whole system ties together!

10.9   Grow and Change Your Identity

Keep celebrating (feeling the joy) and run this new #1 Action until it becomes second nature, i.e. a new Autopilot habit, just as automatic as brushing your teeth.

NOTE: This could only take a very short time, depending upon the quality of your celebrations :) You don't always have to repeat things for many days. Anchoring to existing habits can embed changes rapidly. It's a myth that you must repeat for 30 or 60 days to form a new habit – make it easy and piggyback on an existing habit!

Before long (when you feel ready), you can repeat the design process for your second and third Aspirations that you considered earlier in this chapter of the book.

Then, as you develop your skills even further and your confidence grows, you will start seeing opportunities for improvement, which will make your life easier and happier.

You might even start involving your family and work colleagues, as we will explore further in the following chapter.

The big win is when you change your "Self-Identity".

How you see yourself, e.g. "Yes, I'm a procrastinator, ha, ha..." significantly impacts your behaviours.

This system enables you to change your identity (slowly but surely), and then the associated corresponding behaviours naturally follow.

An example: Imagine your identity fits this statement: "Exercise and rabbit food is not for me". One possible way to change this unhealthy identity would be to start small and Anchor a five-minute (or even two-minute) walk after dinner with your partner. Celebrate these walks, and they soon become a 30-minute walk, and so on, until you develop a healthy habit of a park run every Saturday... Your identity slowly evolves to fit the statement, "Exercise is really enjoyable, and I feel so much better as a result". You are much more likely to choose healthier foods because these New Actions "Fit" your New Identity. You have broken Mental Shortcuts about yourself and rewired new ones.

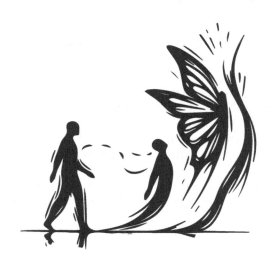

When your identity changes, then massive changes can begin! And yet, we start so small and easy that it's hard to comprehend how significant the change can be in very short periods.

Well done!!! I hope you are starting to see the power and potential of the "Easy" Fit to Care Methodology.

Keep reflecting and embedding these new habits; the world will be your oyster.

10.10 Self Fit Summary

1. Start small, and you can easily make transformational changes to improve your life.
2. Embedded within this introductory programme are the foundations to change your behaviours for good.

   a. Be mindful of your problem areas that you want to improve, i.e. Aspirations
   b. Be creative with the potential Actions that could help, starting with the ones that have the most impact and are most straightforward.
   c. Evaluate carefully to determine your priority Actions.
   d. Design your system to ensure that the priority Actions flourish and become second nature with little effort.
   e. Do not underestimate the power of the Anchor and Autopilot sections – this is where the magic happens, and when actions become tricky – always link back to your Beacons on the Hill.

Practise, and behaviour changes will naturally grow and transform your identity and life.

Remember, it's impossible to fail with this methodology. If you are struggling with an action, scale it down, even if it needs to be a very tiny, effortless action, e.g. tying a shoelace, and then build from there.

Download the file as an overview reminder of the Fit to Care System – keep this handy.

The Meaning & Implementation Methodology

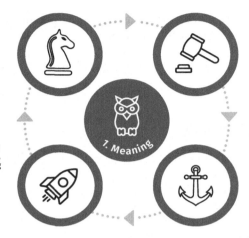

2. Aspiration

Connect Aspirations to what matters, "Meaning" and prioritise the easy wins first.

3. Action

Design the most appropriate Actions that serve your Aspirations.

5. Autopilot

Turn these transforming Actions into Autopilot habits, that make everything so easy.

4. Anchor

Design the most appropriate Anchors that guarantee your Actions.

7. Meaning

If your NHS organisation is already working with us, you can engage with the Fit To Care online community to share experiences, case studies, and what works best. Ask your line manager if they are working with www.FitToCare.co.uk

10.11 Self Fit – Troubleshooting

* A golden rule to remember with the Fit to Care Methodology is that **You Cannot Fail** with this system. Every reflection is a learning opportunity.

If a new Action is challenging or is not happening regularly, be mindful of where the difficulty is:

- Is the trigger/anchor moment not as regular as you first expected?
- Did you forget to visualise the trigger/anchor moment in advance?
- Have you been celebrating? Were the celebrations authentic?
- Did you fail to use the Beacons on the Hill framing if you were in the celebration trap?

Systematically look at your design, step by step, where the problems are.

NOTE:

1. Always start easy. For example, you might have started with an Action of a five-minute walk. If that is seemingly difficult, scale it down to one minute, and if it needs to be, make it EASY so that you can make a start. And don't forget to celebrate, even if it is only one minute! Every new action is contributing to the new you and your meaning in life (Beacon on the Hill) – celebrate this.

2. You might need to revisit your list of Actions (step 2) to see if another Action might be easier. For example, you might have chosen the wrong #1 priority Action. Instead of choosing the phone in another room, we might have kept the dog downstairs and out of your room.

Don't beat yourself up if you make a mistake – learn from it and move on. These actions will help you glean more genuine knowledge, i.e. ALL FOUR of the Ks (Academic, Skills, Viewpoint, and Doing – from Section 3).

10.12 Bonus – Stopping a Bad Habit!

Here is a bonus of a case study around stopping a bad habit.

We've discussed creating good habits, new habits, and new actions. However, you can also use this fundamental system to stop habits. So, here's a real-life case study from my personal experience.

The start trigger was my wife when I asked her, "What would you like me to stop?" Within a nanosecond, she responded, "Stop biting your nails; it drives me crazy." So historically, before I researched this and completed the Meaning Methodology system, I would have said, "Oh, it's fine. You know, it's nothing. It's so insignificant. How can that bother anybody?" And that was my start frame. So, I was in denial and in a state of Pinpointing. It was convenient for me to ignore this. But when I became more aware, I started listening to these cues a bit more. I realised that the environment in the family wasn't as good as it could be. Then, I reverse-engineered the system and applied it to stop a particular behaviour.

So, let's go through it in some detail then. For me, the beacon on the hill was easy when I realised and became aware that my family's love was supreme. So why annoy your other family members when you can do something about it? It's essential, and what you realise when you do fix some of these things is that change can be pretty remarkable. So that's an easy beacon on the hill for this one.

In this case, the Aspiration was easy, too – stop biting your nails, Anthony!

However, the Actions required a little thinking... because I'm NOT doing something – I'm stopping something. So, what's the action to help stop the nail-biting? My high-level reflection was that I bite because I don't like long nails. Okay, Action #1 was to set a time for and complete a weekly nail clip. This would mean my nails would never be long enough to justify nail biting.

How to Anchor once per week? (Remember to match frequency, time, and place.) This was relatively straightforward, too, as I always finish work on the dot at 5.00 pm on a Friday (and start my weekly housework tasks allocated). So, I just bolted on an extra tiny task – clip nails after turning the laptop off at 5.00 pm each Friday (before the chores) – easy. I also visualised the nail clippers at my desk and did the celebrations when I trimmed my nails on a Friday night, so all was good; it was relatively easy to think through and set up.

However, what I found in the middle of week one, after the first nail clipping session, sitting on the sofa late in the evening, watching the last bit of TV drama before bed, and I noticed, because of the self-awareness, was that I'd started just to put that fingernail towards my mouth and started the idea of chewing a nail. What I realised there and then was that I was reacting to tension. So, if I'm ever stressed on a work project, or if there's some tense TV moment, that's another thing for me to go onto Autopilot to bite the nails even though they're already trimmed. So, from that realisation, I set up a second Action, which was if I ever felt like that, I'm going to use a stress ball; the stress ball then becomes a double whammy because it helps to strengthen your hands and your wrists, and at the same time stops you from nail biting. Interestingly, this Action did not have a fixed time slot, e.g. Friday at 5.00 pm – this one only activates in times of tension that can't be predicted or planned. Nevertheless, the tension trigger was a valuable aid to prompt the stress ball to grab! So, I've now ended up having two actions that helped me prevent myself from making this inappropriate nail-biting habit. You can see how it evolved, and that's fine – we are all just learning.

I started with the trim on a Friday and added a second action through my self-awareness. The other thing was the celebration, so I do my celebrations and feel proud of myself. This is a 45-year habit! – "I've done it. I've sorted it."

Together with celebrations from your partner and your family members where they go, "Oh my God, you've done it. That's brilliant!" And it didn't take long, either. I felt this was a done deal before the end of week one and embedded by week two.

I haven't gotten into that bad habit since, so it worked quickly... It was not one of these things you've "got to do for 30 days"; it can happen quickly.

Use the system, do it properly, think it through, be self-aware, and constantly adjust. If things aren't going well – tweak the process. Don't feel pessimistic about failing; new learning takes you closer to success. Hopefully, this case study just added extra context to the system, and you now know that you can use it as a stopping habit and create new ones.

When you have embedded these ideas and skills, and the 4As become easy to recall, you are ready to move forward and explore how to utilise them with your colleagues at work.

Progress with the mindset that there is much we can do to improve your life and the patient experience. Let's start that journey in the next chapter – Team Fit.

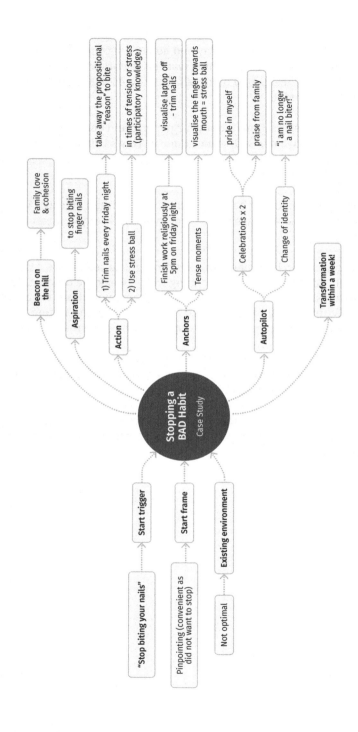

Family love & cohesion

take away the propositional "reason" to bite

in times of tension or stress (participatory knowledge)

visualise laptop off – trim nails

visualise the finger towards mouth = stress ball

pride in myself

praise from family

"i am no longer a nail biter!"

Beacon on the hill

to stop biting finger nails

1) Trim nails every friday night

2) Use stress ball

Finish work religiously at 5pm on friday night

Tense moments

Celebrations x 2

Change of identity

Aspiration

Action

Anchors

Autopilot

Transformation within a week!

Stopping a BAD Habit

Case Study

Start trigger

Start frame

Existing environment

"Stop biting your nails"

Pinpointing (convenient as did not want to stop)

Not optimal

"Nursing is an art: and if it is to be made an art, it requires an exclusive devotion as hard a preparation as any painter's or sculptor's work." **Florence Nightingale**

Together for Tomorrow: Pioneering a New Era for the NHS

Chapter 11

Team Fit

Team Fit Introduction

Now that you have developed the most critical skills and techniques from Self Fit, you can start to develop them with your team.

I believe in the human spirit. We are fundamentally good people, and nobody comes to work to fail. It does not matter what tensions exist in the team; tensions are usual. We will put all that behind us and move onwards and upwards. Our therapy will not be looking backwards at who has wronged us but through **shared Meaning and purpose**. We will heal and thrive in our work through action and making changes for the better. We will achieve, and we will celebrate.

You, as nurses, are in the fortunate position of being closest to the patient. This gives us unique opportunities to be the Patient Champions and facilitate fantastic change within the NHS. However, we will only achieve this if we work together as an authentic, cohesive unit, as a genuinely unbeatable team, and we will.

One key element that will contribute to strong teamwork is the establishment of your team Precepts, which refer to your behavioural norms or the ten commandments that your team lives by. We will discuss these Precepts in detail shortly, but first, let's focus on enhancing our communication and decision-making processes through effective meetings (then we can use these meetings to agree on the Precepts).

11.1 Communication, Decisions and Meetings.

"If someone were to offer me one piece of evidence to evaluate the health of an organisation [team], I would want to observe the leadership team during a meeting." Patrick Lencioni

Lencioni is so right. Section 1 provides evidence of how dysfunctional NHS meetings are; this must be one of our top priorities in our evolving team. We must also ensure that we use our meeting systems to incorporate wisdom through the 4Ks (Academic, Skills, Viewpoint, and Doing knowledge) discussed in Section 3.

Note: We must acknowledge that changing team dynamics, especially meetings, is naturally a significant challenge because most people have fixed mindsets/mental shortcuts and fixed identities about who they are and their role within meetings. Therefore, don't expect change to be immediate or straightforward. However, the systems and tips below will make the change process much easier and more efficient!

The Main Problems with Most Meetings:

- There is insufficient focus on moving forward and solving things and too much emphasis on complaining.
- We don't hear from everyone (4Ks).
- We don't know which opinions are most common and which are outliers.
- Individuals dominate.
- Individuals interrupt.
- Individuals are not present (e.g. mobile phone use).
- Interpersonal issues creating tension.
- We suffer from the four tyrannies:[117]

  - The tyranny of the first response
  - The tyranny of the most passionate
  - The tyranny of the most verbose
  - The tyranny of status

As this list shows, meetings are difficult to manage, which explains why so many are poor.

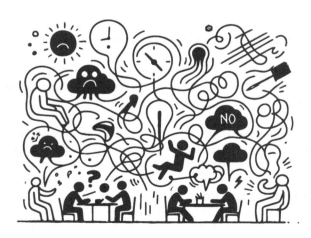

---

117 "The Power of Teams: How to Create and Lead Thriving School Teams" by Samuel Crome

Let's look at a fictitious case study to make the points:

Emily has gathered her team for their weekly meeting and has posed a question: 'We need to discharge five patients this week to hit our targets; how do we do it?' She looks across the table at her colleagues and waits.

She has asked the question 'everyone', and so who answers first is determined, largely, by the personalities in the meeting.

There is a strong likelihood that the first idea mentioned will not represent the aggregated wisdom of the people engaged. Yet, it is often mistakenly taken to be.

We often react to the first answer as if it were correct. We allow it to speak for the team.

That's what happens in Emily's meeting. Pat answers first: 'We should expect more from GPs to manage these patients.' [A handing off of responsibility.]

Emily presumes a tacit agreement with the first answer and quickly moves to problem-solving. 'Okay, what ideas do we have to return these patients to primary care more quickly?'

You can see how easy it is, especially in an overwhelmed environment, to "Pinpoint" and miss a lot of wisdom (4Ks) that we need to make better decisions for both the team and patients.

We need a better system!

11.2   Different Meetings for Different Purposes

We need different types of meetings to deliver different elements of the work. We can be much more efficient and effective if we tailor our meetings. Below is a summary of three different types of meetings I encourage you to consider:

**Type 1 Awareness Sharing (AS) Meetings (incl. Managers) –
Daily 10 mins**

- Share any operational/admin information, e.g. Handovers, events, issue alerts, etc.
- Quickly getting the team onto the same page.
- This can save a lot of time, e.g. with other forms of communication like emails.
- It's also good to build in this human interaction with teammates, allowing you to look out for one another.

Type 2 Team Progress (TP) Meetings – Weekly 30-60 mins

- This meeting is about reviewing team priorities and agreed Aspirations that the team has committed to focus on. It's about the usual business and the best use of resources.
- First, don't plan an agenda upfront. Build a live agenda in the meeting by having everyone share their top three priorities. Members can use Red / Amber / Green to summarise the elements of work they are updating.
- Then, there will be an open debate to agree on the colour status and, thus, the critical focus areas for the meeting.
- These meetings can yield suggestions for Insight and Analysis (IA) Meeting Aspirations (see below).

Note:

- This avoids presentations on things the team doesn't see as important.
- This type of meeting must not be about strategic change, e.g. upgrading a system or part of the pathway – because this meeting has insufficient time to do this justice.

Type 3 Insight & Analysis (IA) Meetings (exclusive to one issue) – As Required 60-90 mins

- This is where we add the most value, have the most fun, and make the most impact!
- Drill into critical issues that significantly impact the patient/service.
- Manage these meetings through the Meaningful Meeting System (see below).

DO NOT combine Team Progress (TP) with Insight & Analysis (IA) Meetings! This common mistake results in neither being done well.

Always remember to cascade critical information to team members who cannot attend the meetings – apply this principle to all three types of meetings.

If the meetings are managed well like this, there will be no such thing as "too many meetings". By getting things right the first time, you always save resources and reduce stress levels. Well-managed meetings are always a good investment!

Team Challenge – Start your 1) Awareness and 2) Team Progress Meetings this week.

Make a start right now. Please take photos of these key pages for your colleagues without the book and share them with the team. Discuss, and hopefully, your teammates will agree to try these new types of meetings.

TIP: Have a meeting about the different meeting types (all three explained) to understand and agree on the concept before attempting to run any of these meetings for real (otherwise, people get confused by too many new things at once). It sounds crazy to have a meeting about meetings, but it's not!

NB The success rate of implementing these changes will be much higher if you all (as a team) go through the programme together. If you are reading this book in isolation, maybe talk to your manager about it and get them to contact www.FitToCare.co.ukso you can all go through the programmes together simultaneously. The online course has video explainers providing more context and examples for each meeting.

11.3 Individual roles within meetings

You can become more sophisticated with the Team Progress and Insight & Analysis Meetings, allocating roles to individuals (that can be rotated from meeting to meeting).

Team Progress (TP) Meetings:

- The note-taker or secretariat is obvious, but what about a "Conflict Miner"? This person looks for tension between team members and can spot who is not opening or showing hostility, e.g. through body language. The Chair can periodically ask the Conflict Miner if any tension needs to be teased out.

Additionally, for Insight & Analysis (IA) Meetings:

- What about a ChatGPT[118] operator that can run queries live in the meeting for extra ideas?
- Another role to consider is gaining all four levels of knowledge with a 4K Role. For someone to constantly evaluate – "What are we missing?"
- *An essential role is the timekeeper to inform people when they have reached their one or two minutes' speaking time* (see the Meeting System below). This is probably the most challenging transition for many people, as you must think carefully about what you need to get across quickly and clearly. Many people don't think things through and "waffle on". Implement these time constraints, and you will be amazed at how quickly your meetings can change and how much more productive they will become.

11.4 The Meaningful Meeting System: Maximise Engagement and Wisdom

Bringing diverse opinions to the table is not enough. How we work "at the table" (physical or virtual) is critical in determining whether we hear and learn from all our perspectives.

This system is for the Insight & Analysis (IA) type of meeting. The intention is to either:

1. Gain a lot of insights and knowledge from a sufficiently broad range of stakeholders. Or:
2. To get agreement and consensus on the Aspiration / Agenda item. However, if it can't be completed in this session, then it will evolve to:
3. Getting agreement and consensus on what actions need to be taken, by whom, and when.

---

118 ChatGPT is an AI (Artificial Intelligence) application that can be accessed online for free (as at time of publication) and can add a lot of support / ideas – even live in a meeting. https://chat.openai.com/auth/login

Agreement and consensus, from a 4Ks approach, i.e. an adequate variety of stakeholders with a range of Skills, Viewpoints, and Doing experience, are critical for these meetings to add the most value.

General Guidelines (not cast in stone):

Pre-meeting:

- The manager determines the "Aspiration" / agenda item for review at the meeting and confirms that it is aligned with the Meaning/ Purpose of the team.
- *[NB The example above was, "We need to discharge five patients this week to hit our targets; how do we do it?" In our new team, we might deem this as NOT aligned with our Meaning because we all know that the implicit implications are that patients will be discharged too soon, which is unsafe, and as Patient Champions, we are not prepared to do this. So, our Aspiration for the meeting might instead be, "How do we optimise our discharge processes and systems?"]*
- The manager considers the appropriate stakeholders that need to attend – with the 4Ks in mind (to optimise the shared knowledge and wisdom of the session).
- The manager determines the meeting roles in advance (these can rotate from meeting to meeting), e.g. Chair, Secretariat, Conflict Miner, etc. NB A Timekeeper will be essential, especially to start with, as keeping within one-two minutes is very difficult for most NHS staff.
- The agenda item and summary context are distributed to the attendees in advance to give them sufficient time to think through and reflect on their views.
- Managers can also use our App, www.fittocare.co.uk/Insight-Genie (see voucher at the end of the book) to gain critical insights before the meeting. This will boost the chances of the meeting becoming a final agreement and ratification process, or reduce the number of meetings required on a particular Aspiration. The App makes Insight and Analysis meetings much more efficient and effective.

General Guidelines (not cast in stone) During the Meeting:

- The Chair describes the initial "Aspiration" and context to the team.
- Everyone gets a turn for every round – 60 to 120 seconds each to make your most salient points per round (e.g. three Likes, three Dislikes, etc.). It's not too long to avoid the tyranny of the verbose. A

short timeframe encourages members to think and prioritise to get the key points across efficiently.

- Members can pass if they want to (but are encouraged in a safe way to contribute).
- No interruptions or comments from other members whilst members are speaking.
- The Chair/manager will summarise all key points and the Team's "direction of travel" after each round.

Round 1 – Clarify: Go around the room in order, with everyone sharing an initial brief 30 seconds with any clarifying questions (e.g. are we just thinking about what's in our control or other departments/ organisations?).

Everyone can and should ask if required.

The manager / Chair will clarify (e.g. everyone involved in the patient's pathway – so all departments/organisations). **NB**, as a rule, the Chair will update after all members have completed the round. However, the Chair should apply common sense and address it immediately if they feel an early question is likely valuable to all members.

The secretariat records the critical points for the Chair.

The Chair summarises and checks everyone is happy to continue. (Not time limited.) These summaries are critical times for the Conflict Miner to look out for unhappy team members and can sensitively ask them to add more insights to the summary.

Round 2 – Like: Go around the room in order (you can change the order, too), with everyone sharing what they LIKE about the Aspiration (e.g. I think this is a great aspiration to work on as there is so much we can do… there are always bottlenecks with XYZ). **NB**, this is a good round for the Chair to evaluate if the Aspiration is likely to be progressed by the team; you could sense from this round and the next that it is not a "goer" from the team's perspective.

The secretariat (note taker) records the critical points for the Chair.

The Chair summarises and checks everyone is happy to continue. (Not time limited.) Again, the Conflict Miner needs to pay close attention to ensure all members are happy with the round summary.

Round 3 – Constraints: Go around the room in order (you can change the order, too), with everyone sharing what they see as constraints / what they are concerned about with this Aspiration (e.g. I am worried that this is still focusing on dysfunctional targets that put our patients at risk…).

The secretariat records the critical points for the Chair.

The Chair summarises and checks everyone is happy to continue. (Not time limited.)

Round 4 – Ideas for Action: Go around the room in order (you can change the order too), with everyone having two minutes to share their ideas for Actions to address/improve the Aspiration (e.g. we need to collect some data to be sure, but I feel that the biggest bottleneck is pharmacy… we need to work with them to provide information early…).

The secretariat records the critical points for the Chair.

The Chair summarises and checks everyone regarding the actions that need to be progressed. (Not time limited.)

Reflection Time: Everyone reflects (e.g. five minutes of quiet time) on what they think should be the priority actions from the knowledge sharing.

Chair's View: The Chair summarises what they view as the key Actions (and why) that should be followed up after the meeting.

NB, some Aspirations will have been agreed upon during this process, and no additional Actions will be required, while others will need many Actions before the team is happy to embrace and own them.

Round 5 – Check: Go around the room in order (you can change the order, too) with everyone to check whether everyone is happy to either, 1) sign off, or 2) agree with the actions. (E.g. happy, but you missed the pharmacy, and I think that should be on the list.)

Chair's Decision: The Chair finalises the Actions list (with explanations for any areas that might be contentious so that the whole team can "buy in").

The Chair then manages the Action owners and delivery timeframes. If managed skilfully, hopefully, there will be volunteers for the Actions and support for one another in the delivery.

During this process, the owners and timeframes are agreed upon – ensuring that owners are happy with both the task allocation and the timeframes given.

Admin: The secretariat tidies up the notes to the meeting and distributes them to the team promptly.

Meaningful Meeting System

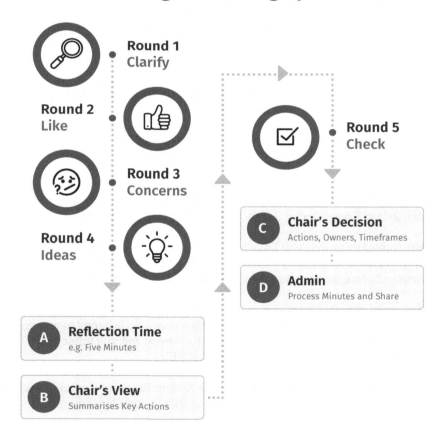

Round 1
Clarify

Round 2
Like

Round 3
Concerns

Round 4
Ideas

Round 5
Check

C Chair's Decision
Actions, Owners, Timeframes

D Admin
Process Minutes and Share

A Reflection Time
e.g. Five Minutes

B Chair's View
Summarises Key Actions

11.5 Run a Team Insight & Analysis (IA) Meeting – A simple challenge

By now, you should have already discussed and explained the three meeting types, and the team should be comfortable with this new concept.

To start your IA meetings, pick a topic that is relatively easy to understand and that members will be familiar with. Start simple so that you minimise possible confusion. The first one enables you to focus on the practicalities of the new meeting system.

For example, the Topic could be "How do we improve on Handovers between shifts?". This topic will be familiar to everyone and is not difficult to understand. However, the meeting could still generate some great insights for the team to consider for improvements.

Follow the guidelines in 11.4.

11.6 Run a Team Insight & Analysis Meeting – Nurse Team Precepts:

The next step, now that the team is familiar with the new meeting system and has already managed meetings like this, is to run an IA Meeting (using the system in 11.4), and the Aspiration for the meeting will be a little more challenging "Team Precepts". I have built a first draft set of precepts for you to provide a draft kick-start; however, the team must own these, and if that means re-writing them, rewrite them (but you shouldn't need to make many changes).

Note: This draft is just to save you time, but if you fear that teammates will feel that "this is being done to them", then a starting point could be to start with the NMC code (see Appendix3) and the agenda item becomes "Let's review the concept of Team Precepts, as we have been advised to, let's start by analysing the NMC Code".

From all the nurse interviews I have undertaken (more than 150,000 words in the transcripts), I believe that these ten precepts (below) are a robust foundation for your team. I feel that these are the general guidelines of a team I want to work within, and I believe that most nurses do, too.

What are Precepts?

Precepts are general rules intended to regulate behaviour or thought, such as "the legal precept of being innocent until proven guilty". They form morals that bind us together with a shared Meaning/purpose and can be very powerful forces within a team.

The 2015 "Rose Report", formally titled "Better Leadership for Tomorrow: NHS Leadership Review",[119] was commissioned to explore and provide recommendations on leadership within the NHS.

Lord Rose highlighted the importance of a shared vision, and the report recommended the creation of a short NHS handbook or passport/ map that summarises the NHS core values in short and/or visual form. This was suggested as a measure to be published, broadcast, and implemented throughout the NHS to ensure that the core values are well understood and integrated across the organisation.

The Precepts are my version of the Lord Rose recommendations.

Nurse Team Precepts for your consideration/adjustment and ultimate sign-off:

1 Identity – Nurses are "Patient Champions".

We are closest to patients; we are the foundation of change and the best resource to make the NHS work and be sustainable.

2 Belonging – Authentic Teamwork.

We respect every nurse, and no nurse is to be left behind. We trust, listen, empathise, and support one another.

3. Adequate Training and Support is a Priority.

We will train and support each other to be professional in all that we are asked to do. Trained so that Professional Autonomy trumps the tick-box. (Ask for a second opinion where we believe guidelines are inappropriate.)

---

119 https://assets.publishing.service.gov.uk/media/5a7f64e9ed915d74e33f628c/Lord_Rose_
NHS_Report_acc.pdf

4. Positive Attitude.

Nurses are the "can-do" members of the NHS. We are action-oriented, adaptable, and calm in the face of adversity.

5. Positive Conflict.

We encourage nurses to challenge where they believe they can add more value to the patient or the NHS. It must be constructive, positive, caring, and sensitive.

6. We might be Wrong.

We are constantly aware that we might be biased and not have all the relevant information. We will consider all four levels of knowledge (Academic, Skills, Viewpoint and Doing). We are always open to listening and reflecting. When in doubt, we will ask for other opinions.

7. Constant Innovation.

We embrace lifelong learning and always ask where we can improve – for patients, saving NHS resources and for nurse self-care.

8. Striving for Great Implementation.

We always consider the optimisation of all initiatives with the Fit to Care Methodology (the right Aspirations, Actions, Anchors and Autopilot).

9. Enjoy Work.

We manage time together in the workplace and are not afraid to have some fun and enjoy each other's company.

10. Celebrate Achievements.

We remember every day why we are nurses and celebrate how much we improve patients' lives.

Team Challenge – Agree on the Precepts using the Meaningful Meeting System:

1. Use the Meaningful Meeting System to process (and change if required) these Precepts so the team can agree on and sign off on "The Nurse Team's Precepts". You must all be happy with them as you commit to working on them in the future.
2. Share the Draft Precepts before your Insight & Analysis Meeting and follow the system.
3. Write up the Precepts and pin them in places where all team members will regularly see them.
4. Use the Precepts to help shape everything you do as a team.
5. In times of challenge, e.g. conflict between team members, return to the Precepts; they will help you resolve the tension and reduce stress levels.

For example, let's go back to one of the quotes in Section 1, where two clinicians were verbally and racially abusive to one another in front of many patients. In this situation, instead of "What do I do?" the manager has a solid platform to resolve such issues quickly and efficiently.

"P2 **We respect every nurse**, and no nurse is to be left behind. **We trust, listen, empathise, and support one another.**

P4 We are action-orientated and adaptable, and we **stay calm in the face of adversity**.

P5 We encourage nurses to challenge where they believe they can add more value to the patient or the NHS. It **must be constructive, positive, caring, and sensitive**.

P6 We are constantly aware that **we might be biased and not have all the relevant information**."

You can see how valuable the Precepts will be in real-life scenarios and how practical they can be to "break frames" and reorient people to become focused on our Meaning again, i.e. the Patient and staff well-being.

11.7   Email Communication/System

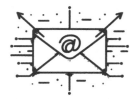

The "Email" System:

Introduce a new email system to the team by first explaining the new system in an Insight & Analysis meeting. This needs to be the theme of the discussion/meeting with your colleagues:

Our time is precious, and we should constantly improve our use processes to improve outcomes/results. Therefore, let's explore a new email system together. There has been a lot of research in this area, and I think we can take a few simple steps to make a big difference for us all and make all our lives easier...

The system elements for us to consider and work on are:

1. Consider and Reflect:

- Do you need to send this email? Will it add value?
- Are you emailing the right person? Is it appropriate to go to them, or are you spamming them? Don't send emails just for the sake of it. Is it more suitable to go to an admin team?

Each situation will be bespoke; often, there is no black-and-white answer – think these things through.

2. Subject Line:

Please make sure that the subject line is short but has these four elements:

(T) **Topic**
(T) **Time** (it will take me to review)
(I) **Importance**
(U) **Urgency / Call to action**

For example (A good example):

Subject: Flu Venues / <5 Mins / Importance High / CTA email by 6.00pm today

Example that will not get read and there will be no response:
Subject: Flu

3. Body Text

Please provide sufficient **background** and details so people can respond adequately, but keep it concise.

Please use **headings and subheadings** so people can read and understand quickly.

Again, **keep the word count as low as possible** for quick review. (Will it fit reasonably onto the screen of a mobile phone?)

Please provide **details of your availability** (before the deadline) so that people can reach you to clarify any details should they need to.

Email System Summary:

Please do not underestimate the power of such a simple email system; it can profoundly impact you. By helping each other in this way, we will save vast amounts of time, get more things right the first time, reduce Workaround and Rework Time, and reduce stress and overwhelm for all.

11.8   Applying the 4As.

Now that you have more efficient and effective meetings and emails, you will generate more appropriate Actions. It's essential to recall what you learned from the Self Fit Programme, i.e.

- Aligned Aspirations: Consider them in your Team Progress and Insight & Analysis meetings and ensure you are always aligned with the Team's Meaning and Purpose [Precepts].
- Positive, make a difference Actions are now much more significant, and we need to optimise their delivery by utilising the Anchors and Autopilot techniques. Apply these techniques for every Action

assigned to every team member, boosting productivity and reducing team stress.

More work on Actions: Sometimes you leave a meeting with an Action that has not been thoroughly analysed and planned. In this situation, you might need to run your own Insight & Analysis Meeting specifically for your Action to get more perspectives from your colleagues.[120] OR you might be able to develop this planning alone through the techniques explained in 10.5 and 10.6.

For every Action, optimise with an appropriate Anchor; see section 10.7 for a reminder of the considerations you should consider (Visualization, Location, Time, Frequency).

And with every Action you should also **invest in Autopilot work, too**. See section 10.8 to recap on authentic celebration, changing identities, and ways to avoid the "don't be such an idiot trap".

11.9   Checklist For Best Practice Teamwork (Above and Beyond the Precepts):

The Precepts will be a very powerful foundation for the team. Better communication through meetings and emails will also be very helpful in reducing stress and overwhelm. In addition, the team should also build the following into their culture:

1. Authentic Care – trampoline listening. 'Overcommunicate' your listening: sit forward, head tilted, give eye contact, nod, give a steady stream of affirmations 'uh-huh, gotcha'. Encourage them to keep going and to give more. Don't jump in to interrupt too quickly.

2. Welcome The Messenger: When receiving unwelcome, challenging, or unexpected feedback, you must 'hug' the messenger and tell them you value it. That way, you can ensure they feel safe enough to tell you the truth next time.

3. Above and Beyond Thank-Yous: When you enter a highly successful culture, the number of thank-yous you hear seems slightly over the top.

---

120 Consider www.fittocare.co.uk/Insight-Genie to help you (see voucher at the end of the book).

However, there is strong evidence that a leader can generate a sense of safety, connection, and motivation by overdoing thank-yous.

4. Design Collisions: Create Collision-prone spaces that allow team members to 'collide'. For example, aligning team members' schedules so they share the same fifteen-minute coffee break daily can have a powerful impact on team connectivity.

5. Cook Bad Apples: in The Culture Code, Daniel Coyle found that a single person can disrupt team life. In a study, a 'bad apple' was planted in teams to undermine the team's work by using body language and words of dissent. It worked, and these teams performed poorly over time. In one team, though, the experiment did not work: this was because one of the other team members used their **warmth and humour** to steer the group back on track. This was all due to this one member's healthy way of managing conflict.

6. Remove Splinters to Avoid Infection: For example, when people splinter off into subgroups, counteract this by restructuring and forming new groups for projects to prevent potential fault lines and reset any cliques that may begin to emerge.

7. Have Fun: Don't underestimate the power of having fun together and finding humour in the day. Social time, such as Xmas or Team achievement nights out, is a powerful way to boost belonging. Laughter is the most fundamental sign of safety and connection.

8. Capitalise on Threshold Moments: For example, when a new staff member joins your team, make sure they feel especially welcomed. Proactively encourage each member of your team to welcome them. Our first experiences have a long-lasting impact on our sense of being part of a team.

9. Negative News Must be in Person: This informal rule is used in many successful team cultures. If you have negative news or feedback to give someone, even negligible, you must deliver it face-to-face. This rule isn't easy to follow, as it's far more comfortable for both parties to communicate electronically. Still, face-to-face communication works better because it deals with tension upfront and avoids misunderstandings.

10. Meeting Etiquette:

- Review the agenda (when you have one) in advance
- Arrive on time
- No mobiles
- Active participation (proper levels too)

11. Work and Present like a Scientist[121]:

We spend too much time thinking in one of these three ways: preachers, prosecutors, or politicians.

- Preacher style = we're convinced we're right and speak 'theory as gospel'.
- Prosecutor style = we're aiming to prove someone else wrong.

In both these approaches: 'I'm right, and you're wrong, and I don't need to / will not change my mind'. We go on the attack to protect our ideas.

Politician style is when we're trying to win the approval of our audience. I might tell you what you want to hear, but I'm probably not changing what I think!

Instead, thinking like a scientist means you **prioritise humility and curiosity over conviction**. Back to Socrates, "All that you know is that you know nothing," don't allow your ideas to become your identity. Look for reasons why you might be wrong, not just why you're right. Listen to ideas that make you think, not just those you like. Always surround yourself with people who can and will challenge your work, not just the ones who agree with your conclusion. Market research with your stakeholders, NOT just in your mind!

Write this list out so that you can keep it as an Aide Memoir:

- Authentic Care – trampoline listening
- Welcome The Messenger
- Above and Beyond Thank-Yous
- Design Collisions

---

121 "Think Again: The Power of Knowing What You Don't Know" by Adam Grant is as follows (Grant, A. (2021). Think Again: The Power of Knowing What You Don't Know. New York, NY: Viking.)

- "Cook Bad Apples"
- Remove Splinters to Avoid Infection
- Have Fun
- Capitalise on Threshold Moments
- Negative News Must be in Person
- Meeting Etiquette
- Work and Present like a Scientist

11.10 Overwhelm TIP – Apply the Jenga Mental Shortcut

Even with these improvements to the Team, which will have a
significant impact quickly, you will inevitably still feel overwhelmed.
To help with this, I want you to remember another very helpful
Mental Shortcut.

Mental Shortcut – Think Jenga

In the game Jenga, you have a structure. That structure has a foundation, meaning you can remove some aspects whilst retaining the core structure and purpose/essence.

From now on, think about your work in the same way. There will be elements that are foundational and others that can be removed. This concept will be a significant element of Patient/Organisation Fit, but I have started to become aware of things now. Note that the things you spend a lot of time on add little or no value to the patient or the team. Start to keep a little notepad of work that you could remove without impacting the patient/Jenga tower!

11.11 Start to value yourselves more.

Nurses are amazing. They blend clinical skills and compassion to provide patient care, educate, guide, and act as guardians in times of crisis. They are critical thinkers and problem solvers who skillfully manage healthcare's complexities. They change patients' lives. Nurses possess a broad array of clinical skills, including gathering health data, administering medications safely, and performing wound care with precision. Nurses are adept at monitoring vital signs, interpreting patient symptoms, and making critical decisions quickly to ensure the best outcomes. They also have advanced skills in operating medical equipment, managing IV lines, and providing life-saving interventions during emergencies. Nurses develop, implement, monitor and evaluate patient care plans, working closely with healthcare teams to ensure a cohesive approach. They educate patients and their families on health management and preventive measures, demonstrating a commitment to holistic care. Nurses' expertise, compassion, and dedication make them indispensable in delivering high-quality healthcare.

I repeat NURSES ARE AMAZING. However, being overwhelmed, stressed, and under pressure can often make nurses feel burnt out and even doubt the profession.

This next task is to remind yourself why nursing is so incredible.

Pocketbook "Positive Log" Task – Patient Impact:

Ideally, please do this as part of a whole Team initiative, i.e. you all do it. Just for a day,[122] log your meaningful interactions with patients. It could be pain relief at just the right time, easing a relative's grief, spotting a doctor's mistake, or not forgetting the two sugars in the tea. What connects you to these other human beings that "emotionally touch" you or the patient?

Make the list.

 Remember why you do this job and the positivity you bring to many lives. Yes, there are tough times (that we will work on together to improve), but let's not underestimate how amazing you are and what a privilege this job is.

At the end of the week, when the whole team has managed to "Positive Log" their day, meet to share some stories and CELEBRATE. Give each other a metaphorical pat on the back; this needs to be authentic – you are fantastic, and so is the job – start to believe that again.

Here are a few ideas for the team to make this an even more significant event:

Awards Ceremony: Host an awards night to honour outstanding achievements, exceptional care, and dedication. Categories could range from 'Best Team Player' to 'Innovation in Patient Care'.

Thank You Notes: Encourage patients, families, and colleagues to write thank you notes or testimonials highlighting the positive impact the nursing team has had, showcasing their importance and contribution.

Public Recognition: Use internal newsletters, social media, or local media to highlight successes and stories of exceptional care within the nursing team, giving them the public recognition they deserve. Managers and Chief Nurses, let's take this seriously and put some effort into building solid Nursing Teams. This investment will pay back many times over.

---

122 If doing as a team – set the team a challenge of doing over a week, to build flexibility in for all team members.

11.12 Reduce Pressure and Stress (A High Impact Month).

Now that we have improved our love of the job and appreciation of each other, let's reduce stress! We have already started this journey by improving meetings and emails, but there is more we can do, and in this next section, I encourage you to make the next month a big one by following these recommendations:

First, think back to the Self Fit Chapter. You determined your Beacon on the Hill. In this work setting, I hope that from your agreed Precepts, your Team's Meaning/Purpose is to be "Patient Champions".

Next, I am suggesting that your first work Aspiration should be to reduce stress and improve nurses' well-being so that you can better serve patients.

Now that you are getting handy with the notebook, spend a few days being aware of all the things that contribute to stress and harm your well-being.

These could be things like:

- As soon as I park the car, I have knots in my stomach, and I fear coming into work.
- I never get a chance to have a drink all day (nurse's bladder).
- I never get a chance to take a break and talk to anyone.
- I never get a chance to have lunch.
- I never leave work on time.
- Etc.

Make your list and then rank the ones that have the most detrimental impact on you that you would love to improve.

At the end of the week, when the whole team has managed to compile their list (and rank order it), set up an IA Meeting (Insight & Analysis Meeting see below and section 11.2 for details) for the team to prioritise the top four Actions (with corresponding Anchors and Autopilot celebrations) that should be worked on. As a team, focus on embedding one per week over the next month.

Meaningful Meeting System

Bespoke to Stress Challenge

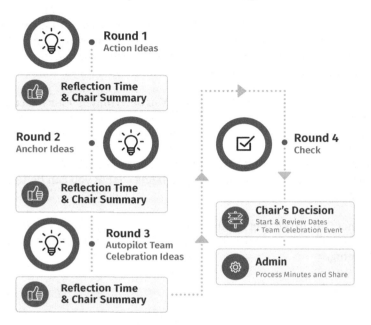

Round 1
Action Ideas

Reflection Time & Chair Summary

Round 2
Anchor Ideas

Reflection Time & Chair Summary

Round 3
Autopilot Team Celebration Ideas

Reflection Time & Chair Summary

Round 4
Check

Chair's Decision
Start & Review Dates
+ Team Celebration Event

Admin
Process Minutes and Share

You can continue this sequence of well-being Actions and support one another for a while, but hopefully, after a month or so, you should see and feel real progress.

For example, let's choose to work through a possible Action that the team might wish to prioritise: "I never get a chance to have a drink."

* The Action might be to drink more and more regularly. (The Aspiration is staff health and well-being, contributing to the Beacon on the Hill. (Being able to perform as a Patient Champion at a high level.)

* The Anchor could be that every time you wash your hands (a well-established existing Action), you will take a drink of water. (Perhaps the team set up a space for water bottles next to the sink?)

* The Autopilot celebration could be a nod to a fellow nurse whilst drinking: "Look, I'm doing it – we've got this".

In a book, it's impossible to prescribe how each team should develop its Actions, Anchors and Autopilots. As explained in Section 3, Combinatory Explosion means doing a "checklist" for you is impossible; trying to be too descriptive would be foolish. This book can only provide guidelines and examples. But the real solutions will come through your unique circumstances and your 4Ks.

Don't forget the details in Self Fit, Chapter 10; there is no such thing as failure, just learning. If the team is struggling with a particular Action, analyse why. You might need to scale back the ambition a little? Redesign the Anchor? Make the celebrations more authentic? Whatever the constraint, there will be a way to improve, and working as a team will make it easier to solve.

11.13 Monthly Reflections

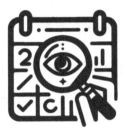

At this point in your team's development, introduce "Monthly Reflections".

Make this part of your Team Progress Meeting. In advance, each team member can think through:

1. What am I most proud of this month? (This is a form of Celebration to help embed the new Actions you have been working on.)
2. What would I like to work on next month? (Focus on Aspirations and Actions to progress and make us feel better, i.e. closer to our Meaning/Purpose.)

Through the implementation of Chapters 10 and 11, you are building the knowledge and skills from an individual level in Self Fit to a Team level with Team Fit, and these are preparing you for the next level of Organisational/Patient Fit.

"To be "in charge" is certainly not only to carry out the proper measures yourself, but to see that everyone else does so too."
Florence Nightingale

Together for Tomorrow: Pioneering a New Era for the NHS

Chapter 12

Patient / Organisational Fit

This is the third level of development, which is more challenging but rewarding. It's all about enhancing your skills as a Patient Champion so you can better understand patient needs and improve Shared Decision-Making. By using the 4As[123] and 4Ks[124], you'll be able to shape your organisation in a way that benefits everyone. You can redesign pathways, use technology more efficiently, reduce Workarounds and Rework, improve patient care, boost your well-being, and make the NHS more sustainable.

Due to word count limitations, this third programme cannot be covered in this book. If you would like to delve deeper into this third level, you can visit our website, www.FitToCare. co.uk, and enrol in our online course with live consultancy support, which can take your organisation to the next level.

---

123 Aspirations, Actions, Anchors, Autopilot
124 Four Layers of knowledge – Academic, Skills, Viewpoint, Doing

Summary and Implementation

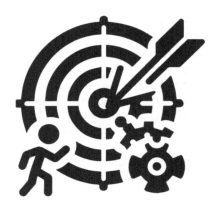

Summary

In the Introduction to this book, I included a table illustrating the key elements of the first Positive Healthcare Revolution. Now, from the analysis of this book, we can complete the table, including the key elements that are required for the Second Positive Healthcare Revolution:

The 1st Positive Health Revolution (Why & What)	The 2nd Positive Health Revolution (How)
Universal Healthcare Coverage	Patient Focus (break the silos)
Government Responsibility for Healthcare	The Nurse as Patient Champion
Free at the Point of Use	Teamwork with creative and critical thinking

1. Patient Focus – Breaking the Silos:

Imagine a healthcare system where patient care is seamlessly integrated across all divisions, breaking down the traditional silos that hinder effective treatment. 'Fit To Care' champions a unified approach where the sole focus of patient well-being drives every decision and action. This book lays a roadmap for transforming care delivery by ensuring that patient needs and holistic care pathways guide every operational and clinical decision, leading to more coordinated and comprehensive patient care.

2. The Nurse as Patient Champion:

This book positions nurses as caregivers and central advocates for patient welfare within the healthcare system. 'Fit To Care' empowers nurses to lead, equipping them with the tools and authority to act as champions for their patients. This ensures that the nurses' unique insights and holistic view of patient needs shape care practices and policies, reinforcing the critical role nurses play in enhancing patient outcomes.

3. Teamwork with Creative and Critical Thinking:

Teamwork in healthcare often follows strict protocols that can stifle innovation. 'Fit To Care' encourages a shift towards a culture where teamwork is infused with creative and critical thinking. This book promotes an environment where diverse healthcare professionals collaborate effectively, bringing together their creative insights and analytical skills to solve complex health challenges innovatively. By fostering a spirit of intellectual curiosity and open dialogue, the book outlines how teams can overcome entrenched practices to achieve exceptional care outcomes.

We[125] believe and have been able to support these beliefs with robust data and evidence that a Second Positive Health Revolution is possible and that the time is right for such transformation.

13.1   At an Academic level, you have what you need.

This book has been many years in the making. It provides everything you need at an Academic level of knowledge to support individuals and facilitate team building that will make a significant difference to you and your patients.

As previously discussed, in our Western culture, many professionals believe that Academic/technical knowledge is all you need.

However, please always keep Section 3 in the forefront of your mind. To approach "wisdom", where real progress is made, you need all four levels of knowledge: Academic, Skills, Viewpoint, and Doing.

---

125 Myself and the nurses who have been interviewed and supported the editing of this book.

Specialists in a particular field spend hundreds and thousands of hours reflecting upon all four levels of knowledge. This enables them to communicate with you and your organisation in a bespoke way, considering your unique scenarios and environments. Specialists can understand your knowledge gaps and likely Pinpoints, Mental Narrowing, and Bias Traps. This is the difference between the Academic knowledge that the book provides and the wisdom that specialists in a particular field can provide.

We all fall into Bias Traps of thinking – e.g. this book is excellent – I can now go off and do it, as I have everything I need. When I have done it, I will be even more 'Fit to Care'.

You can do this in the same way the specialists have, i.e. through years of knowledge gathering at the levels of all the 4Ks.

However, if you want/need to make progress in a matter of weeks rather than years (because even with great intentions, your day job will get in the way, as we all know), then it is advisable to take on specialist support to assist you with the implementation.

I was no different. I love to learn, and I constantly read every book that interests me (and this becomes very tiring for family members). So, my attitude has been to learn by myself for too many years of my career. I was such a lost cause that I even drew my technical drawings for planning permission for a kitchen extension rather than get an architect to do them. Looking back now, this is making me laugh out loud. Yes, it proves that almost anything is possible when you put your mind to something. However, although it was built without a hitch, this approach isn't sensible if you want to get things done quickly and efficiently.

Within recent years, and this has tied in with my insights into Information Overwhelm (remember the chessboard example in section 3), I have realised that how on earth can I even hope to get close to wisdom without the support of specialists in various fields? I can't; they have thousands of hours of experience and wisdom that I can't even hope for because time is finite and precious. Should I spend days and weeks understanding planning permission and how to draw technical plans, or should I let an architect do it (with a much higher chance of planning success) in minutes?

I have now grasped this nettle: **"For every area that I want to excel in, I need to work with a specialist."** From this point onwards, my life and productivity have been transformed.

If it weren't for my Business Coaches, I would not have written this book; it would never have happened. If it weren't for my publisher's support, this book would not be anywhere near as good. Without such support, the book would have taken me years rather than a few months to produce.

I hope this book has given you valuable insights that have taken me years to collect and refine. I also hope you take this last insight to heart: **"When something is important, work with specialists to get it done quickly and efficiently. There are no shortcuts to wisdom."** NB you must still procure the right specialists to avoid disappointment, but the principle is sound!

Nurses need more respect and more support. Nurses are the NHS's greatest asset as they are closest to the work and have so much front line knowledge, and as such are the foundation of NHS wisdom. This knowledgehas to be utilsed more efficiently so that nurses can drive the change that the NHS so desperately needs. Let this book be the catalyst for your change, and don't let this opportunity go to waste.

National Ambition

We believe that this mission of supporting nurses is so important that we aim to support the whole UK. This mission is driven by altruism rather than money; any profits will be reinvested into our organisation to support growth and an even more comprehensive range of support to nurses across the whole of the UK.

Today, we stand at a crossroads in healthcare. Our path must be paved with collaboration and insight, driven by our collective commitment to care. The NHS's potential is boundless, but we must persevere and be courageous. Let us rally together, harness our shared passions, and propel the NHS towards a future of excellence. The time to act is now.

13.2 Next Steps

- Take the Fit to Care Scorecard (next page) and see how you have progressed from your start position at the beginning of the book. If you haven't done it yet - there is no time like the present!

- To assist with your organisational Insights and to make sense of your findings - use our system Insight-Genie – you will be amazed at what you discover from your stakeholders and how easy it is to implement. Take advantage of a free course and a free Genie research report (next page).

If you want to develop further or would like help or more support (Courses, Training / Mentorship), please get in touch with Fit To Care[126]

---

126 https://www.FitToCare.co.uk/contact

Fit To Care
Stop & Question

Want to continually improve your productivity for your stakeholders? Take the Fit to Care Insight Scorecard to identify your productivity baseline.

Discover opportunities for improvement by benchmarking your ability to capture your stakeholders' insights and the effectiveness of your meetings.

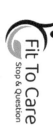

Take your free 5-minute assessment
fittocare.co.uk/scorecard

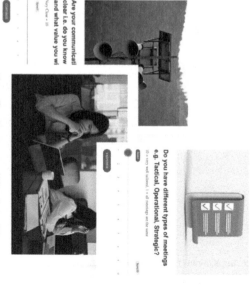

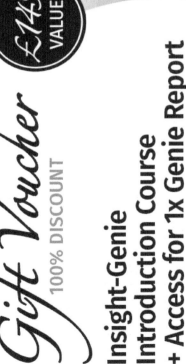

Gift Voucher
100% DISCOUNT

£149 VALUE

Insight-Genie
Introduction Course
+ Access for 1x Genie Report

REDEEM AT
fittocare.co.uk/insight-genie-course

DISCOUNT CODE **CKRC52Z**

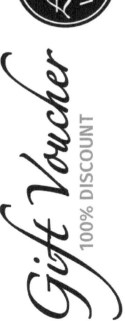

🪔 *Insight Genie*

For further study:

Professor John Vervaeke – Awakening from the Meaning Crisis (YouTube 50 hours of free lectures)

Dr BJ Fogg – Tiny Habits (book)

Professor John Seddon – Freedom from Command and Control (book)

Henry Priest – Biased (Book)

Thank you for reading this book, and we hope to provide you with more educational resources in the future.

"So never lose an opportunity of urging a practical beginning, however small, for it is wonderful how often in such matters the mustard-seed germinates and roots itself." **Florence Nightingale**

Together for Tomorrow: Pioneering a New Era for the NHS

Glossary

Action – Actions that contribute towards your Aspiration(s).

Anchor – is an already automated Action/habit (our Anchor) that you do on autopilot, e.g. you will always flush the toilet "without thinking". Linking a NEW Action to this Anchor will dramatically increase the chances of implementing the new Action.

Aspiration – Goal contributing to your Beacon on the Hill.

Autopilot – The process of undertaking an Action without thinking about doing so; a habit. Unconscious competence. We develop to this state by piggybacking on an Anchor and celebrating when we complete the new Action. This supports the ongoing repetition of the new Action until it becomes second nature, i.e. an Autopilot process.

Beacon(s) on the Hill – The things that are most important to you (linked to Meaning), that you want to continue after you have gone. E.g. your partner or children. Tangible things that you can easily picture in your mind, that you would metaphorically "walk over hot coals" for.

Bias Traps – where the brain has selected a mental shortcut to utilise in a particular situation, but the mental shortcut is inappropriate (e.g. wrong time, wrong place, wrong context). As a result, errors contribute to "excessive Mental Narrowing".

Bullshit / Bullshitting[127] – We can't lie to ourselves but can (and often do) delude ourselves. Here, we use Pinpoint logic to justify a particular decision. "Just one cigarette won't hurt me...". Bullshit illusion accomplished. Here, you have deluded yourself through Pinpointing and the power of "now" to go ahead. As a result, you have fallen into the trap of Mental Narrowing, i.e. not considering that it is never "just one", that what is the damage to your children witnessing this act, just one, will damage your lungs, etc. It's easy to bullshit, especially with a tiny bit of Pinpoint logic. Be extra mindful of this.

Celebration Trap – Beating yourself up for celebrating something that seems insignificant. This is a big mistake, as even the most minor things

---

127 On Bullshit by Harry G. Frankfurt

contributing to your Action, Aspiration and Beacon on the Hill are essential!

Constraint Traps – Where we make assumptions that what we plan to do will work without sufficient Mental Opening to consider all the relevant forces that are likely to stop, prevent, or take our initiative off course.

Easification – Focusing on everything in the system designed to be as easy to think about / do as possible. To reduce Mental Overwhelm, and reduce the reliance upon Motivation (because motivation is unreliable).

Fixed Mental Shortcut – This is where you have used a Mental Shortcut (often successfully over a long period) to such a degree that you can't see another way – your frame has become fixed. So even when this Mental Shortcut is causing Bias and problems, you still can't "Break the Frame" to make a new, more appropriate Mental Shortcut for the new situation.

Gestalt – an organised whole that is perceived as more than the sum of its parts.

Meaning – is what matters to you and is the source of your energy that enables you to act.

Mental Balance is when you are aware of your Mental Shortcuts and evaluate their appropriateness to avoid Bias Traps. You also constantly consider constraints and "The 4Ks" to guard against inappropriate Mental Narrowing. The result is a balance that enables you to interact with the world optimally.

Mental Narrowing – Academics refer to this as reciprocal narrowing, i.e. the more overwhelming the world becomes, the more you narrow down. Narrow in the sense of rejecting information. This rejection of crucial information could result in relying too much on Mental Shortcuts, which are inappropriate biases. Problems result, i.e. you make poor decisions because you do not consider all the relevant information. These poor decisions create a vicious downward spiral of overwhelm, pressure, narrowing, and constant decline.

Mental Opening – the opposite of excessive Mental Narrowing, i.e. you reflect and become aware of bias. You collect the right balance of information, form better solutions, make better decisions, improve results, and reduce stress and overwhelm.

Mental Overwhelm – where the level of data is so vast, it's impossible for the brain to compute and practically manage. (Thus, the brain needs to find summarising patterns, i.e. Mental Shortcuts to operating in the real world.)

Mental Shortcuts – academics call these heuristics. Your brain finds patterns within large data sets and generates "rules of thumb" or mental shortcuts to cope with an overwhelming quantity of data.

Nowness – Where the desire for something is so strong that you get pulled into a state of Pinpointing. This then often leads to us "Bullshitting" ourselves with small elements of logic that don't represent the complete picture.

Pinpointing – This is related to what academics refer to as Hyperbolic Discounting. Where the brain gets you to focus on a very narrow set of information points, e.g. a lion tracking you down. Pinpointing can be brilliant where you are in danger (its original purpose) but can lead to excessive Mental Narrowing and "Bullshit" in the nowness of desire, e.g. inappropriate eating habits. The negative side of the brain's functionality here is exploited by marketers who look to encourage pinpointing, e.g. of chocolate, "go on treat yourself...".

Precepts - general rules intended to regulate behaviour or thought. E.g. "the legal precept of being innocent until proven guilty".

The 4Ks – four levels of Knowledge required for Wisdom (Academic Knowledge / Skill Knowledge / Viewpoint Knowledge / Doing Knowledge (ASVD).) See more details in section 8.2.

Thinking Too Fast – where the brain has jumped to a conclusion too quickly and inappropriately selected a "Mental Shortcut" that is not fit for purpose, i.e. a "Bias Trap".

Workaround and Rework Time (WRT) – where your actions are not considered the relevant factors (often due to Mental Narrowing or Pinpointing), and you get things wrong, e.g. misdiagnosis or an unnecessary referral. Such deficiencies always result in more work/demand for the system as a whole, so the pressure on everyone in the system gets worse, and patient care/outcomes get worse.

About the Author

Introducing Anthony Lawton, a visionary leader in the healthcare industry and the Founder of Fit To Care. With a wealth of experience in healthcare Training and Development, Anthony is on a mission to inspire a revolution by empowering the frontline (particularly nurses, midwives, and allied health professionals) to recognise their value and to amplify their voices.

As a specialist in bridging the gap between frontline wisdom and senior management, Anthony's expertise supports nurses in believing in their worth and being heard. By reducing Workaround and Rework Time (WRT) and waste, improving hospital financial positions, and ensuring correct practices in the patient pathway, Anthony's approach leads to enhanced job satisfaction, reduced stress, and improved work-life balance for healthcare professionals.

With Fit To Care, Anthony's clients achieve many benefits, including career advancement, expanded skill sets, increased confidence, and greater professional recognition. With a remarkable track record of transforming lives and healthcare systems, Anthony's impact extends to enhanced patient care and improved well-being.

As a Chartered Management Accountant (CIMA), Anthony brings a unique blend of financial acumen and healthcare expertise. Through Fit To Care, Anthony collaborates with healthcare professionals, organisations, and decision-makers to create positive, lasting changes in the industry.

His visionary leadership and dedication to empowering healthcare professionals have garnered him the respect and admiration of his peers.

Let Anthony Lawton inspire and enlighten your audience at your next event. His insights, passion, and commitment to transforming healthcare will leave a lasting impact on all who have the privilege of hearing him speak. Together, let's revolutionise the healthcare industry and improve lives.

Contact via Linkedin or through www.fittocare.co.uk/contact

The Nurses Interviewed

A Huge Thank You To The 20 Nurses Interviewed

Below are the nurses who wish to share their names and views on the book:

- **Aysha Badat:** "Fit To Care inspired me to provide an insight of nursing as a leader. Nurses are the heart of healthcare; and just how you can't build a house without its foundations, you can't build a hospital without its nurses. Global health challenges, however, have a massive impact on healthcare services, in particular nurses who work to use their fine art to provide the best care[128]. Strong nursing leadership is, therefore, key to all progress; leadership is not just about titles, positions or flowcharts, but is the ability to influence others by setting a new example." Aysha Badat BSc (Hons) RGNI MSc ACP

- **Debra Holloway:** "This book is about helping nurses to care for themselves and giving them empowerment, it is a welcome addition of tools that nurses can use to enhance the care that they give and strengthen team working." Debby Holloway, RGN, BA (hons), MSc, FRCOG, FRCN

- **Fiona Cramb**: "There has been a lot of change in the NHS since I started as a student nurse in January 1974! The nursing care has changed from a more task approach, with medicine rounds, back rounds, bed-bath rounds to a much more holistic patient or family centred care approach. A lot of this, as with other changes has generally been good, but as with all change there is often a chain reaction that leads some other issues, e.g. impact of staffing and resources etc which may not have been originally foreseen. Such frustrations have been highlighted in this book and I feel privileged to have been able to discuss some of these with Anthony. Talking is very cathartic! I feel a great gratitude to the NHS for being able to fulfil most of my career bucket-list! I have no doubt that Anthony's book with the inclusion of comments from nursing staff in various areas of practice, will be helpful and lead to further

---

128 "Nursing is one of the Fine Arts: I had almost said, the finest of Fine Arts." Florence Nightingale

meaningful discussions from all areas and grades of staff within the NHS and I hope that at least some of the 'frustrations' can begin to be addressed with the self-help or team work." Fiona Cramb BSc, MSc, RM, RN

- **Fran Dunn**: "The NHS and the partner organisations, in Defence, that share the load and aspirations, are world class providers battling changing expectations and experiences of our patients and staff combined with a changing and challenging financial landscape. This book will enable Nurses at all levels to explore and delve into some of the situations that may be both familiar and unfamiliar to give guidance to remaining excellent practitioners in a challenging environment." Fran Dunn RGN

- **Paul Reeves**: "I chose to contribute to this book because I love nursing. All too often, the contribution nurses make to the well-being of people is undervalued. Nurses are having a tough time at the moment, but we carry on caring, tending, coping, and treating. I believe this book will help nurses gain better recognition, help the profession feel better about itself, and reignite its passion for caring." Paul Reeves BEM, MA, BA, RN

- **Sonya Elworthy**: "Reflecting on how our experiences have shaped us as nurses, can be the best way to prepare us for future challenges within the NHS, it also reminds us that the answers are within our own reach, both as individuals and as a profession as a whole." Sonya Elworthy (RGN)

- **Sue Bacon**: "The NHS is an organisation to be proud of, but we must recognise and learn from our shortcomings. Recognise that the population is growing, we are all living longer due to huge improvements in care, and we must adapt. This book is about improving patient care and outcomes, not by directives from above, but by empowering the nursing staff to be the best they can be, helping teams to work better together and giving everyone a chance to influence how care is delivered." Sue Bacon RN.

- **Tara Iles**: "I have had the pleasure of working with Anthony on the national menopause programme with NHS England. I have seen firsthand how he is determined to make a difference, and this book will make a difference in your mindset and your life. I love being a nurse and always remember that the beauty of nursing is that we are in a highly privileged position to comfort people when they are sometimes at their lowest; they are frightened or panicked. We are the first to be present when people enter the world and the last when they leave it. What a responsibility but a huge opportunity to make a real difference and have a lasting impact." Tara Iles, RN, BSc (Hons), MSc, Msc Senior Nurse, Women's Health, NHS England.

- **Teresa Chinn:** "I have been a nurse for over 25 years, and in that time, I have seen so much change within health and care; perhaps now is the time to stop, take stock and look around as we have so many solutions now ... we just have to recognise them." Teresa Chinn MBE RN QN

- **Trevor Hubbard:** "With nearly 40 years' nursing in the NHS, I am still astonished daily by what we achieve despite the increase in pressures that our teams are under. It is now time for the NHS to get some care and attention to bring it, and all who work in it, back to being the envy of the world. Investment isn't just money, it is making the system more efficient, reducing the bureaucracy, embracing technology, and valuing our staff to benefit our patients." Trevor Hubbard: Experienced Senior Nurse and Transformation Specialist MSc PGDip BA RN JP

- **Wendy Norton:** "Nursing is a rewarding career, albeit one of the most stressful. The impact of the COVID-19 pandemic and the ongoing staff shortages have increased levels of work-related stress and reduced job satisfaction for many nursing staff, resulting in many leaving the profession. I hope this book can illuminate current concerns of healthcare staff and highlight the importance of supporting staff well-being to prevent further loss of highly skilled and experienced healthcare professionals." Dr Wendy Norton FRCN; PhD, FHEA; RGN

Appendix 1

Other Countries Influenced by the NHS

Several countries have referenced the UK's NHS as a model or influence in developing their healthcare systems. The principles of universal healthcare coverage, government responsibility for healthcare services and "free at the point of use" have all been influential.

The World Health Organization (WHO) has highlighted the NHS as a leading example of effective healthcare delivery.[129]

Here are some examples of countries that have looked to the NHS for inspiration:

1. **Canada**: Canada's healthcare system is similar to the NHS in its commitment to providing care funded by taxation and free at the point of use. Studies and policy discussions often refer to the NHS when comparing healthcare systems. For example, Marchildon's review of Canada's health system includes a comparative analysis of healthcare models with specific reference to the NHS. (Marchildon, G.P., "Canada: Health System Review," Health Systems in Transition, 2013)

2. **New Zealand**: New Zealand has sought inspiration from the NHS for various aspects of healthcare policy, particularly in the integration of health services and the emphasis on primary care. The structure and focus on public health within the New Zealand health system have been influenced by the NHS. (Cumming, J., "Integrated care in New Zealand," International Journal of Integrated Care, 2011)

3. **Scandinavian Countries**: While Scandinavian countries such as Sweden, Norway, and Denmark have their unique healthcare systems, they share the principles of universal access and public funding with the NHS. These countries often refer to the NHS in healthcare efficiency and equity discussions. (Saltman, R.B., Bankauskaite, V., Vrangbaek, K., "Decentralization in health care," European Observatory on Health Systems and Policies Series, 2007)

4. **Australia**: Australia's Medicare system, which provides universal access to healthcare, shares foundational principles with the NHS. Policy analysis and health system reviews often compare the two systems, drawing lessons from the NHS's experience in providing comprehensive healthcare services. (Duckett, S., "The Australian

129 "The World Health Report 2000 – Health Systems: Improving Performance", WHO, 2000.

Health Care System: The Potential for Efficiency Gains," A report for the Business Council of Australia, 2010)

5. **Taiwan**: Taiwan's National Health Insurance (NHI) system was launched in 1995 and was influenced by the NHS and other universal healthcare systems. Taiwanese policymakers studied various international models, including the NHS, when designing their health insurance system. They aimed to provide universal coverage and ensure equitable access to healthcare services. (Cheng, T-M., "Taiwan's New National Health Insurance Program: Genesis and Experience So Far," Health Affairs, 2003)

Appendix 2

Targets – More Detailed Analysis

To keep the main book as accessible as possible, I have added extra information regarding "the possible dysfunctions of Targets" to the Appendix.

Upon reviewing the interviews with our sample survey of nurses, a striking similarity emerged with the testimonies from the Francis Report. This similarity suggests that the dysfunctions highlighted in the Mid Staffs case are not isolated incidents but rather, unfortunately, prevalent across the entire NHS due to the cultural norms associated with targets.

The Francis Report (Independent Inquiry into care provided by Mid Staffordshire NHS Foundation Trust January 2005 – March 2009[130]) critically addressed the dysfunctional use of targets within the NHS, particularly how an overemphasis on achieving specific metrics could detract from the fundamental goal of providing high-quality patient care. In the recommendations, Robert Francis QC outlined several key points regarding the use of targets:

Balance Between Targets and Patient Care: The inquiry highlighted the need for a balance between achieving targets and ensuring the quality of patient care. It pointed out that while targets could be useful for measuring performance, they should not overshadow the primary focus on patient safety and care quality.

Cultural Change: The Francis Report's recommendations underscored the urgent need for cultural change within the NHS. They advocated for a culture that values patient care over meeting administrative targets. This includes fostering an environment where staff feel empowered and obligated to raise concerns about patient care, even if such concerns might conflict with achieving set targets.

Leadership and Accountability: The report called for more decisive leadership and accountability mechanisms within the NHS. It emphasised that NHS leaders have a crucial role in ensuring patient care remains the central focus. They were urged to ensure that the drive to meet targets does not compromise patient safety or care standards.

One of Francis's key recommendations is enhancing transparency and openness within the NHS. This means being open about when and why targets are not met and ensuring that such situations are viewed as

---

130 https://assets.publishing.service.gov.uk/media/5a7c1b11e5274a1f5cc75d16/0375_i.pdf

opportunities for learning and improvement rather than as a form of punishment. This approach will foster a culture of continuous learning and improvement, instilling confidence in our ability to address these dysfunctions.

Use of Targets: While the report did not call for the abolition of targets, it suggested that targets must be intelligently applied and monitored to ensure they contribute positively to patient outcomes rather than becoming ends in themselves.

Whistleblowing: The recommendations also emphasised the importance of protecting and encouraging whistleblowers who highlight unsafe practices or failures in care, even if these issues relate to pursuing targets.

In essence, the Francis Report acknowledged the role of targets in driving improvements but warned against their misuse. It emphasised that the welfare of patients must always be the paramount concern, with targets serving as tools to enhance, rather than detract from, the quality of care.

Please see specific quotes below from the Francis Report, which can be compared with the quotes from our nurse surveys so that you can draw your own opinions on whether Mid Staffs was an isolated case or whether such targets are driving a culture of dysfunction across the whole of the NHS:

- "The drive to meet the waiting time target had a detrimental effect on staff and on the standard of care delivered. There was persuasive evidence that this even led to attempts to fabricate records."

- "There is no doubt that the pressure generated fear, whether justified or not, that failure to meet targets could lead to the sack."

- "The nurses would go into that meeting and they were told in the meeting that [if] there were any breaches to – that is breaches of the four-hour rule – they would be in danger of losing their jobs. On a regular basis, and I mean a number of times per week, when I was on day shifts, I would see nurses coming out of that meeting crying."

- "I think we were all put under pressure to meet the four-hour target. It wasn't just something that was unique to Mid-Staffs. And there was very much a sense from the SHA, the PCT, Monitor, the Department of Health, that that was a required standard that patients should be able to be clinically dealt with within the department within the four-hour threshold."

- "This evidence satisfies me that there was an atmosphere in which front-line staff and managers were led to believe that if the targets were not met they would be in danger of losing their jobs. There was an atmosphere which led to decisions being made under pressure about patients, decisions that had nothing to do with patient welfare. As will be seen, the pressure to meet the waiting target was sometimes detrimental to good care in A&E. This is inconsistent with the guidance about targets published by DH: It is vital that this target must not in any way jeopardise the quality of clinical care offered to patients..."

- "Another example of the detrimental effect of moving patients to avoid breaches of the target was given by one of the advanced nurse practitioners: I also think that patients were being moved from accident and emergency for whatever reason, to beat the four-hour breach, before they were fully assessed. A good example would be patients who – I can think of an example, perhaps 18 months ago, a patient who came in, very, very ill. Had blood tests done in A&E. I do not think the blood results returned back. He was seen by the basic casualty officer, the most junior doctor. The blood tests were done. As far as I am aware, the blood test results weren't returned for whatever reason. The patient was moved up to the EAU on the four-hour target... and the patient subsequently had a cardiac arrest. I think what happened was the bloods – if they were back, they were not acted on in A&E before the patient was moved out. The patient needed immediate emergency care intervention to prevent deterioration, the deterioration which of course happened when he appeared on EAU. 34. This witness thought that a much more legitimate target would be to aim for access to a consultant in acute medicine within two hours of admission to A&E, a target which had recently been introduced internally."

- "The pressure is alleged to have led to some staff being complicit in the falsification of records in order to make it look as though the target had been met."

- "The pressure of meeting the waiting time target led to practices which were detrimental to patient care."

- "The observations quoted above are examples of something that is of concern about the role of Director of Operations, as she perceived it. She gave the Inquiry the distinct impression that she focused on working with specific issues, such as targets, rather than taking a broad overview of the work of the organisation. While this may be inevitable to some extent in this role, this may have contributed to, for example, the development of an unquestioning target culture."

- "A former staff nurse and whistleblower expressed views about the impact upon targets during the period in which the hospital was making its application for FT status. She said that Monitor was visiting the hospital, and there was real pressure on not breaching the four-hour target (in A&E), so people were actively bullied and pressured into lying about timings. The view of a nurse manager in emergency care was that applying for FT status was the main cause of the Trust's problems."

Appendix 3

The Precepts

The draft for nurses (Chapter 11) offers a comprehensive framework to enhance patient care and the professional environment for nurses within the NHS. These Precepts and the NMC's Code (see below) share common values and objectives, focusing on patient-centred care, professional development, teamwork, and ethical practice. Below is the "Compare and Contrast" analysis of these Precepts with the NMC's Code:

Comparison:

Patient-Centric Approach: Both the Precepts and the NMC's Code prioritise the interests and safety of patients. The precept of nurses being "Patient Champions" aligns with the Code's directive to put the care and safety of people first.

Professional Development and Support: The Precepts emphasise adequate training and support, reflecting the Code's requirement that nurses maintain their skills and knowledge for safe and effective practice.

Teamwork and Collaboration: The Precept of "Authentic Teamwork" echoes the Code's call for collaborative work, respecting the contributions of all healthcare professionals to ensure the best outcomes for patients.

Openness and Honesty: Both frameworks advocate for transparency, with the Precepts encouraging nurses to admit biases and the Code mandating openness and honesty, including admitting mistakes.

Continuous Improvement: The Precept of "Constant Innovation" and the Code's emphasis on reflective practice and professional development aim to continuously improve patient care and professional practice.

Contrast:

Identity and Advocacy: The Precepts uniquely highlight the nurse's identity as "Patient Champions" and agents of change within the NHS. This perspective complements the Code but is more explicitly articulated in the Precepts.

Positive Conflict and Challenging Guidelines: While the Code promotes professionalism and trust, the Precepts specifically encourage positive conflict and challenging guidelines when nurses believe improvements can be made, offering a more explicit framework for advocacy within the profession.

Enjoyment and Celebration: The Precepts explicitly mention enjoying work and celebrating achievements, which are not directly addressed in the Code. This inclusion underscores the importance of a positive work environment, recognising contributions, and enhancing job satisfaction and morale.

Methodological Approach to Implementation: The Precepts introduce a specific methodology ("Fit to Care Methodology") for optimising initiatives, which is not found in the NMC's Code. This suggests a structured approach to implementing changes and improvements in practice.

Comprehensive Autonomy: The Precepts advocate for professional autonomy beyond compliance with guidelines, encouraging nurses to seek second opinions when necessary. This is a more explicit articulation of professional judgment than what is detailed in the Code.

Overall, the precepts build upon the foundation of the NMC's Code, adding depth to nurses' identities and roles as agents of change, emphasising teamwork, innovation, and positive work culture and providing specific strategies for implementing improvements. These precepts complement the Code by enriching the professional and ethical framework nurses are expected to engage in, enhancing patient care and the nursing profession within the NHS.

The NMC Code[131]:

1. Prioritise People

You put the interests of people using or needing nursing or midwifery services first.

---

131 Nursing and Midwifery Council (NMC). (2018). The Code: Professional standards of practice and behaviour for nurses, midwives and nursing associates. NMC. Available at: https://www.nmc.org.uk/standards/code/

You make their care and safety your main concern, ensure their dignity is preserved, and recognise, assess, and respond to their needs.

2. Practise Effectively

You assess needs and deliver or advise on treatment or give help (including preventative or rehabilitative care) without making unwarranted demands on people's time and resources.

You maintain the knowledge and skills you need for safe and effective practice.

3. Preserve Safety

You act without delay if you believe that you, a colleague, or anyone else may be putting someone at risk.

You make sure that you have the right knowledge, skills, and experience to safely deliver each aspect of your practice.

4. Promote Professionalism and Trust

You uphold the reputation of your profession at all times.

You declare issues that might create conflicts of interest and make sure they do not influence your judgement or practice.

5. Respect Confidentiality

You treat information about patients and clients as confidential and use it only for the purpose for which it was given.

6. Work Collaboratively

You work cooperatively within teams and respect the skills, expertise, and contributions of your colleagues.

7. Be Open and Honest

You act with integrity and are open and honest, admitting mistakes and taking whatever action is necessary to resolve any harm caused.

8. Maintain Clear Professional Boundaries

You do not take advantage of your role as a nurse or midwife to form inappropriate relationships with patients or their families.

9. Stay Informed and Reflective

You reflect on your practice and acknowledge any limitations in your knowledge and competence.

10. Engage in Professional Development

You take responsibility for your own learning and development through continuous reflection and updating of skills.